# THRIVE

A guide to optimal health & performance through plant-based whole foods

by
**Brendan Brazier**

**THRIVE** - A guide to optimal health & performance through plant-based whole foods
by Brendan Brazier

Oceanside Publishing
119 - 17 Fawcett Road,
Coquitlam, BC
Canada  V3K 6V2
www.oceansidepublishing.com

Edited by: Bruce Cole
Cover Design: Ryan Mah
Interior Design & Production: Randy Ellis

ISBN 0-9735967-3-2
Printed in Canada

# Table of Contents

FOREWORD . . . . . . . . . . . . . . . . . . . . . . . . . . . . . . . . . . . . . . . .5

ABOUT THE AUTHOR . . . . . . . . . . . . . . . . . . . . . . . . . . . . . . .9

INTRODUCTION . . . . . . . . . . . . . . . . . . . . . . . . . . . . . . . . . .11

CHAPTER ONE: STRESS - THE MODERN PLAGUE . . . . . . . . . . . .14
• Treat the cause, not the symptom . . . . . . . . . . . . . . . . . . . . . .18
• Don't break it if you can't fix it . . . . . . . . . . . . . . . . . . . . . . . .19
• Our 'sickness treatment' system . . . . . . . . . . . . . . . . . . . . . . .21
• Change is stress, adapt slowly . . . . . . . . . . . . . . . . . . . . . . . .22
• Mind-body connection . . . . . . . . . . . . . . . . . . . . . . . . . . . .23
• Optimal balance . . . . . . . . . . . . . . . . . . . . . . . . . . . . . . . . .24
• Be sure not to jeopardize health in its pursuit . . . . . . . . . . . . . .26
• Natural light, daily . . . . . . . . . . . . . . . . . . . . . . . . . . . . . . . .27
• Darkness, for improved sleep and recovery . . . . . . . . . . . . . . . .28

CHAPTER TWO: FOOD'S CONNECTION TO STRESS - AND RELIEF . .29
• Natural or borrowed energy? . . . . . . . . . . . . . . . . . . . . . . . . .29
• The vicious circle of poor nutrition and how to break it . . . . . . . .30
• Appetite will diminish as quality of food improves . . . . . . . . . . . .32
• Increase energy through conservation, not consumption . . . . . . . .33
• A 25-hour day? . . . . . . . . . . . . . . . . . . . . . . . . . . . . . . . . . .36
• A lean muscular body - a mere by-product . . . . . . . . . . . . . . . . .38
• Improve health by meeting nutritional needs, not exceeding them . .40
• Recalibrate the body for increased energy . . . . . . . . . . . . . . . . .41
• In spite of or because of? . . . . . . . . . . . . . . . . . . . . . . . . . . . .42
• To care for your environment is to care for yourself . . . . . . . . . . .44

**CHAPTER THREE: KEYS TO CREATING A BIOLOGICALLY YOUNGER, LEANER BODY** . . . . . . . . . . . . . . . . . . . . . . . . . . . . . . . . .46
- The hormone factor . . . . . . . . . . . . . . . . . . . . . . . . . . . . . . . .47
- Exercise . . . . . . . . . . . . . . . . . . . . . . . . . . . . . . . . . . . . . .48
- Hydration . . . . . . . . . . . . . . . . . . . . . . . . . . . . . . . . . . . .48
- Food - it becomes you, literally . . . . . . . . . . . . . . . . . . . . . . .49
- Which foods are best? . . . . . . . . . . . . . . . . . . . . . . . . . . . . .50

**CHAPTER FOUR: NUTRITIONAL PROGRAM OUTLINE** . . . . . . . . . . .52
- Alkaline advantage . . . . . . . . . . . . . . . . . . . . . . . . . . . . . . .52
- How more plant-based foods can help performance . . . . . . . . . . . .55
- Help your body help you - have a nutritious shake daily . . . . . . . .56
- What a nutritious shake should contain . . . . . . . . . . . . . . . . . .57
- Why timing of nutrition matters . . . . . . . . . . . . . . . . . . . . . .58
- Maximize recovery before the workout even begins . . . . . . . . . . .59

**CHAPTER FIVE: FAVOURITE FOODS** . . . . . . . . . . . . . . . . . . . . . .61

**CHAPTER SIX: SAMPLE MEAL PLAN AND RECIPES** . . . . . . . . . . .79

**CHAPTER SEVEN: STRATEGIES FOR SUCCESS SUMMARIZED** . . .92

**CHAPTER EIGHT: THE STORY BEHIND VEGA** . . . . . . . . . . . . . . .94

**AFTERWORD** . . . . . . . . . . . . . . . . . . . . . . . . . . . . . . . . . . . .104

**APPENDIX** . . . . . . . . . . . . . . . . . . . . . . . . . . . . . . . . . . . . .105

**REFERENCES** . . . . . . . . . . . . . . . . . . . . . . . . . . . . . . . . . . .109

# Foreword

You are very lucky to have this book in your hands. Professional Ironman triathlete Brendan Brazier is a man who walks his talk and lives what he preaches. The information he shares with you in this book strikes at the very heart of the major health problems faced by North Americans today. While we have just about conquered infectious disease, we still battle epidemics of cancer, diabetes, heart disease, autoimmune disease, osteoporosis and arthritis. More than ever before we as doctors have to deal with increasing numbers of people suffering from chronic fatigue and mental illness.

As a medical doctor, practicing what is called 'complementary' or 'integrative' medicine, I have been helping thousands of people over the past 25 years with something called nutritional stress, the most underestimated cause of suboptimal health.

What is nutritional stress? It's the average North American diet, high in refined carbohydrate and unhealthy fat (burgers, fries, fast foods, sugared cereals, soft drinks, chips, candy bars, chocolates). This diet is also too low in complex carbohydrates, fiber and essential fatty acids found in whole grains, legumes, seeds, nuts, fruits and vegetables.

Frequent consumption of fast/convenience foods leads to many problems including food allergies. These allergies lead to cravings for more and the allergy-addiction cycle is established. Over time, the standard American diet (SAD) wears down the endocrine system and our organ reserves. Micronutrient deficiencies develop unless the individual supplements with vitamins, minerals and other important food factors. Psychological, emotional and financial stressors will amplify the nutritional stress and the next thing you know, the victim is taking antidepressants like Prozac, Paxil, Zoloft and others (to the tune of over $10 billion per year in sales).

If you add to this a heavy consumption of other essential nutrient robbers such as coffee, tea, alcohol, cigarettes and drugs, the endocrine system becomes chronically stressed. This leads to high cortisol levels, high blood pressure, blood sugar control problems, high blood fats, especially cholesterol and triglycerides as well as obesity. The immune system is also severely affected leading to recurrent infections and serious conditions such as Chronic Fatigue Syndrome, Fibromylagia and Candidiasis.

The good news is that the effects of nutritional stress can be reversed through a combination of a more alkaline forming, plant-based diet as well as some effective whole food nutritional supplements. Every major epidemiological study concludes that those who consume animal products, including fish (mostly contaminated with mercury and other cancer causing chemicals), milk, dairy products and chicken eggs, have significantly higher incidences of heart disease, cancer, diabetes, arthritis and osteoporosis.

Organic or not, studies show that meat eating is associated with greater morbidity and premature death. People who follow mostly a plant-based diet can run into problems if they rely too heavily on dairy products and wheat and do not eat a large variety of different vegetables, fruits, legumes and other low gluten whole grains. This approach is effective for not only elite athletes like Brendan Brazier but also for anyone interested in improving their health status.

It is also an established biochemical fact that all disease, especially cancer, heart disease, diabetes and arthritis exists in an acid medium. All animal products, refined foods and most high gluten grains create an acid condition in the body. Plant-based diets create more of an alkaline body pH.

The meat-based low carbohydrate or 'cave man diet' advocated by many high-protein diet gurus often does more harm than good because it creates an acid body pH and often a diseased state, termed ketosis. It is therefore not uncommon to see patients with celiac disease, Crohn's disease or candidiasis who have been on long-term meat-based diets suffering from the side effects of excess acid: greater fatigue, muscle wasting and dehydration. A common symptom of candidiasis is constipation, a nuisance worsened by meat consumption, organic or otherwise.

The high protein, low carbohydrate diet may well be in vogue today but it will soon be a passing fad just like many other diet crazes of the distant, forgettable past.

One of the standard but erroneous criticisms of plant-based diets is its purported lack of iron. There is no evidence that vegetarian women who have stopped eating red meat are developing more iron deficiency. In my practice, the opposite appears to be the case. The majority of women who suffer from anemia eat red meat on a regular basis. It might surprise you to know that the best sources of iron are vegetarian, including kelp, brewer's yeast, blackstrap molasses, wheat bran, pumpkin seeds and sesame seeds.

Another mistaken belief is that vitamin B12 is only available in animal foods. Recent studies have shown that some sea vegetables contain substantial amounts of vitamin B12, much more than enough to meet the nutritional needs of anyone. The sea vegetables include arame, wakame and kombu. Other natural food supplements which are rich in vitamin B12 are Blue Green Algae, Chlorella, Barley Green and Spirulina. Vitamin B12 is manufactured by the body's friendly colonic bacteria so supplementing with lactobacillus acidophilus is yet another way of getting vitamin B12 into the body.

Other than cold-water fish, many of which are contaminated with either mercury or polysyllabic carcinogens, omega 3 fatty acids are best derived from plant sources like flax seed oil, seeds, nuts and legumes.

According to numerous studies quoted in books like John Robbins' Diet For A New America and May All Be Fed, it is impossible to create a protein deficient diet provided adequate calories are consumed. Vegetarians who suffer from fatigue, weakness or lightheadedness are most likely not taking in enough calories to meet their needs rather than suffering from a protein deficiency.

As proved by Brendan Brazier, some of the world's top endurance athletes eat only plant-based foods. There is absolutely nothing in animal based diets that cannot also be found in plants. I think that after reading this book, you will no doubt be convinced that a plant-based whole foods diet is the true future of optimal health.

Zoltan P. Rona, M.D., MSc
Medical Editor
Encyclopedia of Natural Healing (Alive Books, 2002)

# About the Author

Told from the onset that 'it won't work', Brendan remained optimistic. Attempting a plant-based diet in the hopes of improving his athletic performance, Brendan's nutritional journey began at the age of 15.

Initially, 'they' were right—it didn't work. Several months of chronic hunger, the need to constantly eat and a decline in energy culminated with a high level of fatigue and ultimately a decline in athletic performance. Told by many that it was a 'common sense' problem with a simple solution; 'do what you did before the problem started, go back to eating meat'—something many athletes resort to after a realization such as this.

If not for his stubborn curiosity, Brendan too would have most likely gone the 'tried and tested' route. From that point on, however, Brendan dedicated himself to find a way to make a plant-based diet work. After years of research and study, trials and tribulations, not only did his findings work, but they worked better than he had ever expected.

That was 15 years ago. Since then Brendan has gone on to be regarded as one of the top professional Ironman triathletes in Canada and is well on his way to international success. Brendan credits his plant-based, nutritional stress reduction diet as a significant reason for his ability to compete professionally in one of the world's most demanding sports.

As a result of Brendan's success, he has garnered a reputation as an innovative cook and recipe developer of performance enhancing plant-based creations. Filled with uniquely original health-promoting recipes, Brendan's full-length cookbook will be released in 2006.

Speaking throughout North America, Brendan continues to teach the value of a properly implemented plant-based diet for improved vitality and performance.

Also, as an advocate of efficient and sustainable agriculture, Brendan encourages the support of companies who employ organic and non-GMO farming methods. Brendan believes that personal wellbeing is intimately connected to environmental health.

Athletic or not, Brendan's 'nutritional stress reduction program' can help you eliminate overall stress to get the most out of life, all while looking and feeling great!

# Introduction

A s a professional endurance athlete, my number one job is to create stress—then deal with it. That's it. I stress my body, allow it to recover, and then do it again. It's really that simple.

Where this can get problematic is in finding balance between these two synergistic extremes: training and recovery. Training is really nothing more than taking advantage of our body's ability to heal itself. When faced with post-exertion muscle damage, the body will surmise that it must grow stronger to perform the task more efficiently next time it is called upon. Really, the body is taking the easy way out; it's easier for it to grow stronger now to reduce the strain placed on it next time it must perform. Little does the body know, as soon as it demonstrates its improved strength, more demand will soon be placed upon it.

What is it that allows some athletes to improve at an exceptional rate, while others become stagnant or make only modest gains? The answer lies in the recovery index (RI), the rate at which recovery transpires. Learn how to speed the RI by means of proper nutrition and lifestyle strategies and improve faster. The ability to speed recovery doesn't stop there. Improved immune function, increased energy level, a reduction in body fat and signs of aging are a few other attributes to be gained by speeding up the recovery process.

If, for example, following a workout I am able to recover quickly, the amount of time I am highly stressed is considerably shortened, enabling me to train again sooner. Over the course of a few months, the extra workouts that this quick recovery has facilitated will significantly improve my fitness. The same principles that I practice to accelerate my recovery from physical stress can be applied to a wide variety of stresses, thereby reducing them as well.

An important fact to be cognizant of is this: the body's response to stress is the same, whether it be the physical demands of sport, the strains of breathing impure air, poor diet or the hectic pace at which most of us now live. A full, productive life will undoubtedly be a catalyst for an elevated stress level. Stress slows progress and therefore it must be minimized for us to reach full potential. Success at anything starts with the ability to effectively cope with stress.

Our bodies are not equipped to deal with many of the modern day requirements placed on them; they simply have not evolved to effectively cope with our increased demands. Can you believe that in the 1950's it was thought that as our technological advances continued, we wouldn't need to work anymore? The theory was that by the 90's, computers would 'serve' us; a romantic ideal that obviously didn't come to fruition. As most of us know all too well, our lives are a non-stop dance from one task to another. The average North American works more now than ever before, and that amount continues to increase as we 'progress.' But work is just one stressor.

Increasingly, more people cite demands of social life and family obligations as 'more stressful than work.' This combined with diminishing air and water quality, and increasingly less nutritious food due to over farmed-fields, leaves us as a culture that is chronically stressed.

There are two ways to deal with these problems. One is to reduce the amount of all-encompassing stress. A reduction in work will do this, but obviously a decline in productivity will result. Both this method and an increased recovery period are effective, but obviously not welcomed by high achievers. As you will discover, a more viable solution is to curtail the effects of stress by implementing an 'uncomplementary' stress reduction program—simply put, improving your diet.

When I first started searching for ways to enhance my athletic performance, nutrition was one area that I investigated. At the age of 15 I experimented with a plant-based diet for the first time. Told from the beginning that it was a bad idea, I decided to find out for myself. 'To be successful as an athlete you must eat meat', this was, and still is the view of many. Of course, as I found, there is simply no basis to support that notion. It is simply misinformation. In fact, I will go one step further and say this: not only has not eating animal products for the last 15 years not stifled my athletic performance, it has significantly elevated it.

Over the course of those 15 years, I have developed a nutritional stress reduction program that has enabled me to improve at an extraordinary rate. Learn these principles, incorporate them, and thrive.

The first edition of *Thrive* was launched in September 2004. I'm pleased to say that the response has been overwhelming. In just five months *Thrive* become a Canadian bestseller.

Having just completed my Canadian book tour— with new ideas still fresh—I decided to make additions to *Thrive*. Therefore, instead of just reprinting, I expanded upon the first edition by adding 32 pages. This second edition includes the following new sections:

- *Change is stress; adapt slowly*
- *Increase energy through conservation, not consumption*
- *Improve health by meeting nutritional needs, not exceeding them*
- *Recalibrate the body for increased energy*
- *Maximize recovery before the workout even begins*

This edition also includes an expanded version of the *Favorite foods* chapter and the *Alkaline advantage* section, plus nine new recipes and the story behind how and why I formulated Vega, a unique plant-based whole food meal replacement. In addition, an appendix listing products that I use—complete with contact information—has been included.

# Stress - The Modern Plague

Simply put, stress is anything that causes strain on the body, regardless of its origin. The sources of stress are many; anything from pollutants in our drinking water, job dissatisfaction, poor nutrition, relationship concerns, over-exercising to under—exercising, are all forms of stressors.

As with fire, when controlled and used by us for a purpose, stress can serve us well. Yet, unbridled, it can consume us. In amounts that our body is capable of adapting to, some stresses are beneficial. Exercise, for example is a stress. Exercise then rest and the body will grow stronger. However, now more than ever, stress has become a real threat to our health and livelihood, often overwhelming us, and in some cases, even controlling us. To suggest it's out of hand is an understatement.

Commonly accepted as one of the leading causes of illness, stress has been shown to precipitate many forms of disease. It's easy to say, 'Reduce the amount of stress in your life and you'll be healthier.' While this is generally a true statement, it's advantageous to 'select' your stressors; cultivate the beneficial ones and eliminate the unbeneficial. All stressors can be classified into three basic categories: uncomplementary, complementary and production.

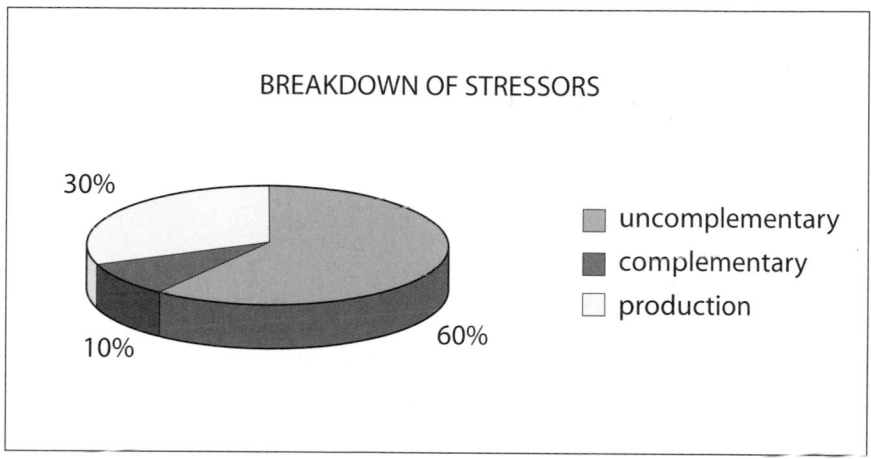

## UNCOMPLEMENTARY STRESS

Produces no yield, should be eliminated or reduced as much as possible, as there are no benefits to this type of stressor. Examples include poor nutrition, worrying about things that we have no control over, setting unattainable goals, poor planning, and environmental (toxins in the air, sunburn)

It's estimated that as much as 60% of the average North American's total stress can be categorized as 'uncomplementary.' Now, 60% is a huge number, especially considering the debilitating characteristics of uncomplementary stress, with no payoff to its host. Within that 60% it's estimated that roughly 70% of that can be attributed to nutritional stress.

This includes the consumption of overly processed foods and foods grown with chemical pesticides and herbicides, as well as an inadequate supply of vitamins, minerals, enzymes, high-quality protein, fibre, essential fatty acids and good bacteria (probiotics). It also includes the overeating of 'empty' foods and the under-consumption of nutrient-dense whole foods that support biological function, activity level and regeneration. Consistently eating acid-forming foods is also a culprit.

By eliminating or greatly reducing nutritional stress, the cause is being addressed, therefore symptoms cannot materialize. Symptoms include poor sleep quality, excess body fat, low energy levels, weakened immune system and lack of mental clarity.

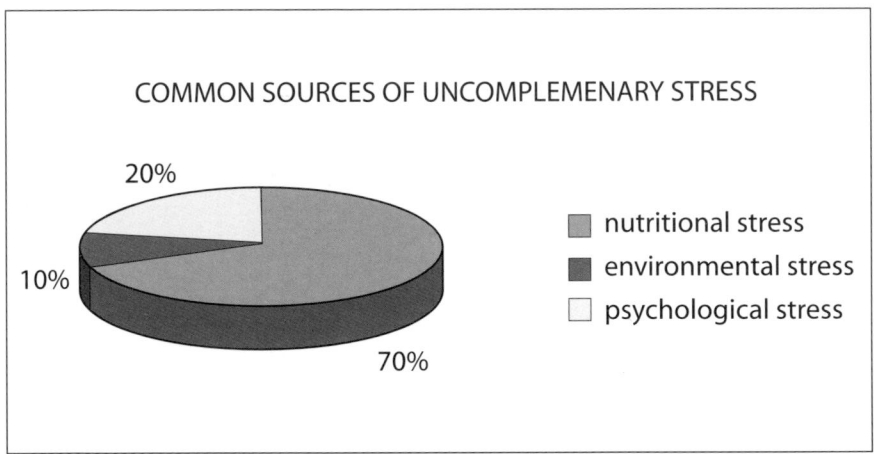

## COMPLEMENTARY STRESS

The right amount of stress to instigate growth and stimulate renewal within the body. The right balance of exercise strengthens us, both mentally and physically, once we've recovered from it. Exercising the optimal amount (which is determined by your ability to recover and deal with other stresses) will strengthen the body as a whole. Gains to be expected include improved muscle tone, a reduction in body fat, increased strength-to-weight ratio, improved immune function, a clearer thought process, and better sleep quality. Exercise essentially creates a 'complementary circle.' It activates the natural healing and regeneration process of the body.

*It is interesting to note that those who exercise regularly are literally younger than those who don't (and they look it). Of course, we have no control over our chronological age. However, our much more relevant biological age is ours for the reducing. When exercised, the body must regenerate its cells more rapidly than when idle. Depending on activity level, six to eight months from now our bodies will have regenerated nearly 100 per cent of their tissue at the cellular level. It will literally be made up of what we eat between now and then. The body of an active person is forced to regenerate rapidly, therefore it is comprised of more recently produced, younger cells—literally a younger body.*

## PRODUCTION STRESS

A wise and necessary way to stress yourself to yield a positive payoff. Examples are physically demanding training sessions for an athletic competition, working overtime, working on personal and family problems, and taking a calculated risk.

This book is not about withdrawing from stress. It's about reducing the uncomplementary variety, harnessing the power of complementary while coping with production and making it all work FOR us, not against us. It is not realistic or even desirable to remove all stress, specifically self-imposed production stress.

Production stress is, as the name implies, an unavoidable by-product of a productive life, a necessary part of modern-day success. For me, it's at times an unhealthy amount of exercise that must be done in order to improve as an athlete. For others, it might be working long hours to complete a high-stakes project, stressful at times, but necessary to achieve a goal. Production stress can be seen as a fun, challenging part of life, with a rewarding payoff. Just by viewing it that way will reduce its negative impact.

*By applying the nutritional stress reduction methods in tnis book, the following benefits can be expected:*

- *Reduced biological age*
- *Increased life expectancy*
- *Loss of body fat and lean muscle maintenance*
- *More energy (without coffee or sugar)*
- *Increased strength and endurance*
- *Improved productivity*
- *Improved mental clarity*
- *Improved quality of sleep*
- *Reduced quantity of sleep required*
- *Improved resistance to infection*
- *Quicker recovery from exercise*
- *Fewer sugar cravings*
- *Desire to excel*

## TREAT THE CAUSE, NOT THE SYMPTOM

A common practice in our society and western medicine is to treat the symptom while neglecting the cause. In traditional eastern medicine, the body as a whole is assessed, as well as the emotional state of the patient. This practice clearly views the person as a complete entity, with the physical and emotional intertwined, dependnt on all its systems to function as a whole. In contrast, traditional western medicine will zero in on the ailment, isolate it, and attempt to fix it.

This can be both a logical and illogical approach, depending on the situation. If, for example, a person breaks his arm skiing, it makes perfect sense to single out the break, set the bone, allow it to heal, and be done with it. Yet, a similar approach is often used with less satisfactory results when dealing with symptoms such as obesity, lack of energy, fatigue, chronic sickness and even wrinkled skin.

A culture's traditions often influence an individual's habits; as a result many of us have become 'symptom treaters.' Look no further than the infiltration of coffee shops. Coffee has become more than 'an enjoyable drink', it has become a necessity to get through the day. 'I can't function before my coffee', or, 'I need a pick-me-up to get through the afternoon.' These notions are the norm in our hectic work world.

Stress is often the cause, yet it is seldom directly addressed. As is usually the case, adrenal gland function can be singled out as the hardest hit part of the body, resulting from repetitive stress. Once the adrenal glands have become fatigued due to the over-production of the stress hormone cortisol, noticeable signs manifest. Fortunately, with the understanding that fatigued adrenal glands are the root of these problems, all of them can be resolved simply by controlling stress and helping to nourish the adrenals, not treating each ailment as an independent problem.

Optimum adrenal health is imperative for optimal overall health. Maca, a South American root vegetable, is my favourite adrenal tonic. An adaptogen that nourishes and strengthens the adrenals, maca is an ideal 'modern world' food to help us manage stress. Detailed information about maca is available on page 64.

*Lesson: Find the cause of the problem.*

## Don't break it if you can't fix it

As mentioned earlier, stress breaks down the body to varying degrees. This is fine; it's how we grow stronger, at least once we recover from it. Provided that we have the resources and know-how to facilitate recovery, this process is healthy. If you don't have them, it can be detrimental.

For example, when a computer tries to download material from several sites at once, the delivery of all information is slowed. Similar to a computer in that respect, the body can only deal with so many demands placed on it. To overwhelm it is to slow the delivery of all results. Unlike a computer though, the body has the ability to prioritize. For instance, if you have a viral infection such as the flu and decide to weight train, the time required for you to recover from your workout will be considerably longer than normal. The reason: the body perceives the viral infection as more threatening as a whole than the acute damage of muscle tissue. Since the body must repair the muscle tissue to at least some degree, the flu will also linger slightly longer.

Another example of our body being good at prioritizing is in the case of low serum calcium. Calcium has a much larger role than just building and maintaining bones. The body utilizes calcium to perform many vital tasks, including playing a part in muscle contractions, nerve transmission, optimizing pH levels, and assisting in heart beat regulation. If dietary calcium becomes insufficient, serum calcium levels will soon follow. As the body realizes this, the vital tasks calcium has been assigned within the body cannot be ignored. For survival sake, if calcium is not available, the body will pull it from the bones. If the body were not equipped with this prioritization mechanism, people with low levels of calcium in their diet would have much greater problems than brittle bones.

As nicely demonstrated by our body, it's not in our best interest to take on projects that ultimately slow our progress. I use this blueprint when designing my training program. Work on one aspect, become proficient, and then move on to the next.

An obvious parallel can be drawn between the 'phasing' training approach and that of common life. If, for example, you are going through a stressful time at work, are just recovering from the flu, and have recently moved to a new city, it's not a good time to start training for a triathlon.

*Lesson: Don't take on more than can be handled. Prioritize.*

## Our 'sickness treatment' system

Our heath care system could more appropriately be referred to as a 'sickness treatment' system. Basically, the medical community treats sickness rather than striving for health. Obviously, the reason we have to treat so much sickness is because we don't care for health. When was the last time you went to your doctor when everything was fine? Doctor's jobs are to help sick people, not to encourage a healthy lifestyle.

If you have to turn to a doctor for the majority of ailments, health has already been breached. That's when the symptom-treating pharmaceuticals start flowing. Drugs can help people; I'm not disputing that. Take people who have high blood pressure, for example. Give them the correct pharmaceutical product, and their blood pressure will be reduced almost immediately, possibly saving their life. If it comes to the point, however, of having near morbidly high blood pressure, mistakes have been made in the past. Yes, it's true a synthetic drug is the best way out of this jam. Of course the best approach would have been to not let the problem develop in the first place. Some people seem to abuse themselves believing that drugs will alleviate the problem when it inevitably manifests. They don't realize that a drug is not a cure. It is merely a relief from a symptom, brought about by a preventable cause.

Don't get me wrong; doctors do us a great service by helping us out of situations that we've gotten ourselves into. It's not the doctor's responsibility to check up on us weekly to insure we're eating well and controlling our stress levels. So, if not just for yourself, do the over-worked medical system a favour and take responsibility for your health.

*Lesson: Your health is in your hands.*

## Change is stress; adapt slowly

There are several reasons why many people struggle with change. In fact those who make positive changes are more likely to discontinue them than those who make negative ones. The reason for this is that those who see themselves as making a sacrifice to try and achieve better health want their investment to pay off quickly. If results aren't nearly instantaneous, interest quickly dwindles. In addition, negative initial results are almost certain to be a deterrent. As described, it's difficult to maintain a person's interest in a healthier diet if it 'doesn't work' right away.

Any physical deviation from routine will be perceived as stress. Even if the change is a positive one, the body must first adapt. For example, if a person has smoked for many years, then decides to quit, the best way is to gradually reduce the amount of nicotine in the system, that's why the patch was invented. It slowly weans the person off smoking's addictive properties. By applying this methodology the chances of success are greatly improved, simply because withdrawal stress is reduced.

A 'New Year's resolution' approach is usually not effective and can quite possibly be counterproductive. To realise that it is actually easier, therefore less stressful (and in effect healthier), to continue to smoke, can seem contradictory to logic. More stress will actually be incurred for a smoker who instantly quits than the one who does so gradually and continues to smoke but at a reduced rate. Of course over time the body will adapt to the stress of withdrawal, overcome it and be healthier as a result; the point is, it does take time.

The same applies to nutrition. When a new way of eating is adopted, the body must adapt. Most commonly referred to as detoxification, this adaptation phase is the body's way of eliminating toxins accumulated over years of poor quality food consumption. Our bodies are equipped with coping mechanisms that allow them to function optimally relative to the nourishment supplied. Seemingly counterintuitive to most people, the first few days of an optimal diet may not be a pleasant experience. Commonly, years of less-than-ideal eating practices have rendered the body nutritionally stressed. The poorer the quality of the previous diet, the longer the detoxification process will last. Those converting from a Standard American Diet (SAD), for example, to an exclusively whole food plant-based diet will likely take in excess of six weeks to 'cleanse' the body of toxins. Common detoxification symptoms may include headache, bloating, diarrhea, nausea, fatigue, and sleep disturbances.

In addition to fibre, any other nutrient that allows the body to excrete toxins and purify the blood such as chlorophyll will require an extended adaptation phase. Chlorella in particular, due to its high concentration of chlorophyll, will help cleanse and detoxify the body.

Implemented gradually, a chlorophyll rich diet can help cleanse the liver, thereby helping to reduce withdrawal symptoms. Those who aspire to quite smoking or eliminate drinking alcoholic or caffeinated beverages will benefit from the gradual reduction of toxins in the liver. Chlorophyll rich foods will help extract liver toxins more quickly, thereby reducing the time in which withdrawal symptoms linger. It's important to remember, along with this detoxification process come the cleansing symptoms. As a sign to back off, severe symptoms are a clear indication to reduce the rate at which change is implemented. The worse a person feels initially simply means there is more to be gained.

*Lesson: Gradual improvement has a better chance of becoming permanent.*

## MIND-BODY CONNECTION

During World War II, wounded soldiers were usually taken to a make-shift medical facility for treatment of their injuries. Many of them were in great pain. Under these conditions, the doctors would inject the soldiers with morphine as a form of pain management until they could be taken to surgery. A common occurrence during these times was for the morphine supply to run out. If a new supply of the painkiller had yet to arrive, doctors were called on to be creative. Knowing about the placebo effect, doctors would tell the soldiers that they were receiving an injection of morphine to numb their pain. In reality, the soldiers were given nothing more than water. Generally, the effect was not as good as morphine itself, but it did help take the edge off the pain. The soldiers expected to be relieved from their pain once given the 'morphine,' so to some degree they were.

The opposite is also true: the effect the body has on the mind is compelling. However, it's often not as obvious, yet can more readily have negative effects. If the body is being stressed beyond a point from which it can reasonably recover, thinking will be altered. Brain chemistry, affecting mood and general outlook, becomes distorted when the body is stressed. I've certainly noticed this effect after weeks of high volume training. Thinking, the ability to reason and cognitive aptitude in general becomes impaired.

*Lesson: Reducing physical stress can improve mental clarity.*

## Optimal balance

When I speak of balance, some people may mistakenly assume that I'm suggesting, 'If you eat good food, it makes sense to eat bad food too.' Or perhaps they twist the intended meaning to justify other actions, such as, 'I've been patient with my co-workers all week; let's see how they like a little balance.' However, when I speak of balance I am referring to balance of positive things. As victims of our cultural common sense, most of us believe 'if some is good, more is better', and 'if lots is bad, a small amount must also be bad.'

Let our body lead the way with yet another example. A small amount of stress is necessary for life; an excessive amount could end it. The right amount of dietary protein will assist in the regeneration of muscle tissue and provide the amino acids necessary to contribute to the construction of a strengthened immune system. Too much protein will dehydrate and place a strain on the kidneys. The appropriate amount of carbohydrates will provide us with readily available energy. Too much will cause a stress response within the body.

Optimal health is about balance. However, optimal performance is not. To be a serious competitor in any demanding sport requires that health must occasionally be overlooked. There are times when the line between sickness and health becomes fine, very fine. The threat of sickness and injury is often overruled by the desire to excel. When I'm at my fittest, nearing a major race, I'm also at my most vulnerable; my immune system has become depleted. A priority becomes the avoidance of any and all possible viral-catching situations. I pretty much keep to myself during these times. Even the slightest contact with a person hosting a virus could spread through my system with the greatest of ease.

If this high level of training is maintained past the point of what is necessary for competition, sickness is likely to develop. With proper precautions, a healthy athlete is able to train at an unhealthy level a few times throughout the year, in the name of performance. That's the nature of high-level sport. It's during immune-compromised vulnerable stages, as described here, that optimal nutrition is paramount. It is literally the difference between sickness and health.

Those who train the most have an elevated risk of infection due to a compromised immune system. We now know that. Interestingly enough, those who exercise the least (such as not at all) are also likely to develop a compromised immune system. This is an example of how a health-boosting activity can get out of hand, compromising its original intention.

If health is your goal, then exercise will most certainly be a component of your routine. It might surprise you to learn that a small amount of exercise is all that is needed to achieve optimal health. Light resistance training with weights one day; up to an hour of aerobic exercise the other, three of each spanning the week; that's healthy. Much beyond that is in the name of something other than health—fitness perhaps, or just enjoyment. Of course I'm not suggesting that you exercise only to the point of what's healthy; that's no fun. Just be cognizant of the fact that health must be achieved first, fitness second so the body can handle the demands. For those of you who aren't as big on exercising, that's fine, no problem; health can be optimized on just a small amount.

*Lesson: Balance of nutrients and exercise contribute to overall health.*

### BE SURE NOT TO JEOPARDIZE HEALTH IN ITS PURSUIT

My mother was once told that she should drink eight glasses of water a day to be healthier. As it turned out, this was bad advice. Yes, being properly hydrated promotes health, but in her case, the stress from worrying about drinking that many glasses of water outweighed the potential health benefits proper hydration could offer. It became such a 'big deal' for her to drink that much water, an additional problem had been created while the original one remained.

You'll be happy to know that this story has a happy ending. My mother discovered that she likes drinking water from a sport bottle. It turns out the problem wasn't the water; it was drinking it from a glass that was the objectionable part. She now drinks eight stress-free bottles a day.

Be cognizant of the 'cost of health.' If you are on a program that is so rigid, and inhibiting, are the benefits being over shadowed? Having to carry and remembering to take numerous pills several times a day, having to stick to your exercise program regardless of all that unfolds around you, is it healthy? Often out of habit, routine, or just stubbornness, ironically health—and therefore performance—is compromised in its pursuit.

If all else is equal, happy people are healthier people. Even the perfect exercise program will not be beneficial if it's not enjoyable. To squeeze yourself into a routine that breeds contempt will counter any positives that it can possibly offer.

*Lesson: Happiness is essential for optimal health.*

## NATURAL LIGHT

Exposure to natural light is essential for optimal health. Some consider natural light a nutrient, as vital for well being as certain dietary requirements. When natural light enters our eyes, the endocrine system becomes involved, helping to maintain our nervous and immune systems.

Vitamin D, also known as the 'sunshine' vitamin, is synthesized in our bodies when exposed to natural light. An essential component for calcium absorption and utilization, Vitamin D is best obtained from natural light.

With limited exposure to natural light, and with conventional indoor lighting as the dominant source, it's possible, even likely, to notice a decline in mood. As you can imagine, once mood declines, most everything else is sure to follow.

Craved by our cells, natural light instigates the production of serotonin, a hormone that makes us feel good. Those with adequate serotonin production commonly have a reduced appetite and a more relaxed demeanour. Once serotonin production drops, depression, weight gain (through increased appetite) and 'cluttered thought patterns' are common.

Personally, I make sure to expose myself to natural light as often as possible, which is easy when training volume is high. However, in the off-season, which is also the dreary winter, I notice a decline in energy unless I make a concerted effort to spend time in full spectrum light.

However, as with many things, some is good but more is not better. Once adequate light exposure has been met, be sure not to allow overexposure of direct sun. Sunburn causes free radicals to be created within the body. As our environment continues to 'evolve' the sun's UV rays have intensified. When significant time will be spent in direct sunlight, it's advantageous to cover up with breathable, natural fibre clothing.

*Lesson: Make an effort to get daily natural light exposure, but not too much direct sun.*

## DARKNESS, FOR IMPROVED SLEEP AND RECOVERY

Melatonin is a hormone that is produced in the pineal gland. Its release is dependant upon the amount of light our body is exposed to. As light fades towards the end of the day, melatonin is released. Soon after its release, melatonin helps prepare the body for sleep by reducing alertness and slightly lowering body temperature. I have found that my ability to get a good night sleep is closely tied to allowing melatonin to be naturally produced. For at least an hour before bed, I make a concerted effort to limit my exposure to light.

For those of you who have trouble sleeping, despite a nutrient-rich diet and even though you employ stress-curtailing strategies, I recommend meditation. Starting about an hour before bed, make sure all lights are dim, just sufficient for navigation. Melatonin will then be released, helping to clear the mind of linear thought, causing the day's events to be blurred. Sit comfortably with eyes closed, breathe with slow, controlled, full breaths and let the mind wander. If melatonin is doing its job, structured thought will be difficult, which is the plan. I generally do this for about 20 minutes, then go to bed and slip into a deep sleep.

Melatonin is also a potent antioxidant. Harnessing its power not only evokes a deep, regenerating sleep, it also speeds recovery at the cellular level.

*Lesson: Darkness before bed will improve sleep quality and recovery.*

# Food's connection to stress - and relief

## NATURAL OR BORROWED ENERGY?

In the afternoon, about 3pm, lunch has started to wear off, and hunger and fatigue is creeping up. At this point, how often do people either have a cup of coffee, a snack high in refined carbohydrates, or both? Coffee and refined carbohydrates give a short energy boost but stress the body. I view coffee drinking as a form of credit, similar to shopping with a credit card. You get energy now that you don't actually have, then you pay for it later. When the 'bill' comes it might keep you down for a few days (unless you drink more coffee to put off the inevitable - kind of like paying off one credit card with another). You'll most likely pay a high interest rate as well, needing more time to recover than if energy was not 'borrowed.' I'm not suggesting you should never drink coffee, but I do suggest that you have some only when you really need a short term boost. Just be willing to allow yourself some extra rest later to compensate for it.

So, what should be consumed as an alternative to provide energy and mental clarity? The answer is a properly balanced snack that contains ample protein, high quality fats, and fibre.

This will not cause inflammation, elevated cortisol levels, or an insulin spike. It will also sustain energy levels for much longer. A good meal replacement drink is ideal in this situation. A full spectrum of nutrients in a convenient, easily digestible form will contribute to building a healthier more vibrant body, one that will not be dependant on caffeine or sugar.

Daily consumption of maca will eliminate the need to 'borrow' energy. As a highly nutritious whole food with the ability to naturally regulate hormone levels, maca improves energy and stamina. In contrast to many so-called 'energy providing' foods that stimulate the adrenal glands, maca is not a stimulant. It's a health-promoting whole food that nourishes the adrenals. Simply put, maca promotes health and healthy people have more energy.

When supplied with many vitamins and minerals, the body will be properly fuelled. Therefore, it will not require as much food. As a result, its hunger mechanism will signal that it's no longer hungry, making fat loss easier.

Here's another fact about coffee: it causes cortisol levels to rise, which lowers the immune system, making the body more vulnerable to infection, eventually leading to body fat being stored. Simple carbohydrates cause an insulin spike that will also cause an elevated cortisol level.

Excessive consumption of coffee and refined carbohydrates can also result in inflammation, a key cause of premature aging. A reduction in inflammation-causing foods will keep the body looking younger longer. Contrast the common mid-afternoon snack of coffee and a muffin with either Vega or my nutrient-rich shake recipe containing maca and chlorella (page 87). Unlike coffee and highly refined carbohydrates which deplete the adrenal glands, my nutrient-rich shake actually helps nourish and strengthen them. The nucleic acids in chlorella also assist in the repair of cellular damage, not precipitating it as coffee does. Of course, the shake also hydrates the body's cells, whereas coffee dehydrates.

*Lesson: Replace refined carbohydrates and caffeine with whole food nutrition.*

## THE VICIOUS CIRCLE OF POOR NUTRITION AND HOW TO BREAK IT

Chronic poor nutrition will leave the body feeling un-energetic and the mind un-ambitious. Conversely, when supplied what it requires, the body will respond with an elevated performance level and an improved mood;

seems straightforward right? The problem is that nutritional stress is often created in the body unbeknownst to the owner, simply due to a lack of knowledge. The common affliction of nutritional stress, all too often creates a vicious circle.

When not provided the nutrients it requires to function optimally, the body tries to 'self-medicate.' This stage begins in the form of cravings. The brain will crave sugary or starchy foods for the sole purpose of elevating serotonin levels. Serotonin is a chemical released from the pituitary gland in the brain. Once released and flowing freely, serotonin elevates mood. A brain chemistry fluctuation such as the release of serotonin has a powerful effect on our demeanour as a whole. Chronically low levels of readily available serotonin can lead to ailments such as clinical depression. Those who have a regular supply of serotonin being released feel better, therefore are more productive and have a lower 'perceived' stress level. When cravings for sugary or starchy food crop up, they are most likely an attempt by the brain to help it 'feel' better. To give into these cravings will satisfy the brain in the short term with its serotonin hit.

The problem is twofold; one, to have to cater to your brain's cravings is not a pleasant way to live—although many now just accept cravings as 'part of life'—and two, by eating sugary foods at your brain's request, insulin levels also rise. Elevated insulin levels cause cortisol levels to increase, which is a stress response. As with any stress placed on the body, elevated cortisol levels can be blamed for a reduced quality of sleep, inability to concentrate, and elevated inflammation which leads to premature signs of aging and slowed recovery from exercise.

This little trick that our body can play on us to help it feel better is merely a 'band-aid' solution. Giving into cravings such as these perpetuates the vicious cycle. The source of the problem is rarely addressed, for any other reason than lack of understanding of nutritional requirements. Conversely, other stresses can precipitate food cravings, the vicious circle works both ways. Many people crave sugary, starchy foods when they've had a bad day at work, didn't sleep well, or are just tired.

> *The most effective way to permanently break the cycle is to reduce uncomplementary stress by eating a nutrient-rich whole food diet; one which contains sources of easily digestible protein, fibre, whole grains and vegetables as a low glycemic form of carbohydrate, essential fatty acids from nuts and seeds, along with vitamins and minerals.*

*Lesson: A nutrient-rich diet will eliminate sugar cravings.*

### APPETITE WILL DIMINISH AS QUALITY OF FOOD IMPROVES

Many parents tell their children, 'Don't eat too close to dinner or you'll ruin your appetite.' (Isn't that the very idea of eating—to ruin one's appetite?) Their motivation behind this of course is to ensure their children 'fill up' on the right kind of food, not empty calories that most unsupervised kids gravitate toward.

Food quality plays a major role in obesity. This serious health concern is never desirable, but it does serve a purpose. It is a clear message that something is out of balance. As discussed earlier, for optimum health and lasting benefits, the cause of the problem must be addressed, not the symptom. Food cravings, usually for sugary or starchy foods, are a telltale sign that the diet lacks nutrients. Cravings and chronic hunger, if not addressed, will lead to weight gain and fatigue in the short term. Long term, any number of heath problems can be attributed to lack of dietary nutrients.

Understudied, this concept actually took some time to figure out. Eat more and food cravings will subside. Sounds simple enough, but it's not so in some cases. As it turned out, a group of racehorses living in a stable together nicely illustrated this conundrum. Since the stakes of horse racing are high, the horses were pushed hard daily in training. This particular stable of horses, a successful bunch, had an impressive track record. However the trainers noticed an odd new habit the horses had adopted. All the horses had, within the same week, stared gnawing on their stables.

Their trainers didn't know what to make of this peculiar behaviour. It was initially thought that the horses must need more food. More food was fed to them, but the gnawing continued, plus now the horses were over-weight! Gnawing continued to the point of the stables looking as though a family of beavers lived there. Weight gain also worsened. The horses no longer looked like racehorses, but rather a bunch of draft horses.

After much deliberation, it was finally determined that the grain being fed to them had been grown in over-farmed soil, therefore lacked essential nutrients. When a new source of nutrient-rich grain was found and fed to the horses, their appetite quickly dropped off and the gnawing stopped. The horses' constant need to eat, their chronic hunger, was actually due to lack of nutrition, not lack of food.

Lack of nutrients in our food is unfortunately common today. As nicely showcased by the racehorses, cravings and the need to eat more food in general will certainly mean the consumption of 'empty' calories, leading to weight gain.

You've probably heard it said before: 'It's not what you eat that's unhealthy it's what you don't eat that is.' This saying aims to inform by suggesting that it's okay to eat some unhealthy food as long as you get your nutritional requirements through the consumption of nutrient-rich ones.

*Lesson: A nutrient-rich diet will reduce appetite.*


## INCREASE ENERGY THROUGH CONSERVATION, NOT CONSUMPTION.

The nutritional value of food as stated by the 'label claim' is of course per-taining to what is in the food, not what the body actually gets from it.

A more sensible way to assess the energy providing attributes of food is to consider its net gain. The net gain of food is the term given to what we are left with once the food has been processed for energy by the body. We all know that the body gets energy from food in the form of several nutrients. However, the more energy the body has to expend to digest, assimilate and utilize the nutrients in the food we give it, the less we are left with.

Quite often I am asked how I am able to gain and maintain strength, lean muscle and have an abundance of energy for high performance training while eating only plant-based foods. Of course there are many factors, as discussed in this book but it's largely to do with choosing food with the 'net gain' concept in mind rather than the conventional calorie counting method.

An example would be the consumption of white bread. Have you ever eaten at a restaurant that served French bread before the main course? In the old days I would wolf down the bread. My stomach would be physically full, yet I would still be hungry. Since white bread is basically void of any useful nutrients, my body wanted to continue eating despite the fact that my stomach was full. To digest, assimilate and then eliminate the white bread requires a large energy expenditure. As a result, the net energy gain from it is very low. In fact, if the bread is buttered or if a trans-fat containing spread is added, the result can actually be a net loss!

In today's hectic, fast-paced world, we are inundated with nutrient deficient foods. Consumed mostly for convenience sake, processed and refined foods have led us to a decline in health and elevated medical costs. Having to consume more of them to 'fill up' due to their absence of usable nutrients, yet high sugar and calorie counts, we have become an obese, energy depleted society.

Back a few years in my more conventional thinking days I would try to gauge my caloric intake requirements based on my activity level and body weight. Eating about 8,000 calories on heavy training days, as determined by my calculations, I would usually need a rest day soon after. I realize now, a large part of my need for the extra rest day was not just to recover from the energy expended during training, but primarily from the energy expended digesting all that food! At the time I would eat lots of starchy, high carbohydrate foods such as conventional pasta and bread. Roasted nuts, usually in the form of peanut butter, would also be a large part of my high calorie yet low nutrient diet. As these are hard for the body to digest and assimilate and have little to offer in terms of nutrients, I was actually robbing myself of energy with every bite.

By consuming more easily assimilated foods a large amount of energy can be conserved. There are two main reasons for this; the first being that the nutrient-rich easily digested foods can be assimilated with less expenditure, and the second is that when more nutrient-rich foods are present in the diet, the body does not have to eat as much as if it were fed 'average' foods. As a direct result, not as much needs to be eaten and therefore digested. This is a huge net energy gain, to be spent as you please. If the body is left to decide, it will likely choose improved immune function and quickened restoration of cells damaged by stress—essentially, 'anti-aging' activities.

Once I realized the value in nutrient density, assimilation, and absorption of food, I began eating in terms of net gain, with no adherence to calorie consumption guidelines. Instead, I focus on consuming nutrient-dense, easily assimilated foods. As a result my recovery rate has significantly improved. I no longer need an extra day to recover from eating copious amounts of conventional food. Enhanced by simple means of increased efficacy, my body now pools its retained energy resources to more quickly recover from muscle damage associated with training. Today, I consume about 30% fewer calories than I did just two years ago yet have more energy—by means of conservation, as opposed to consumption.

Instead of feasting on common refined foods, I now consume whole foods almost exclusively. Raw, alkalizing, enzyme-intact, living foods have become the foundation of my diet. Switching my main carbohydrate source away from refined starches to whole fruits and vegetables was my starting point. In doing so, the majority of my energy needs, obtained from primarily carbohydrate, were now being met by a wide variety of fruit and whole grains.

Raw nuts and seeds, with an emphasis on hemp and flax, as well as legumes supply me with protein and essential fatty acids. The majority of vitamins and minerals I require come from fresh, raw vegetables – dark leafy green ones in particular.

Hydration is also much easier to maintain when more whole, raw foods are consumed over their dry, processed, cooked counterparts.

Specifically, foods that offer a superior net gain are:

- alkaline forming, high in chlorophyll
- rich in enzymes, raw and alive
- rich in pre and probiotics
- best consumed in liquid form

*Lesson: If you don't spend it, you still have it. Think in terms of energy conservation when it comes to vital body functions such as digestion and assimilation.*

## A 25-HOUR DAY?

Stress raises our cortisol levels. Elevated cortisol levels inhibit our ability to sleep. Lack of sleep further raises our cortisol levels. See where I'm going with this? Yes, a vicious circle. Yet, despite having a bad side to them, vicious circles can also get us out of a bind as quickly as they get us into one. Fix one problem, the other will be taken care of, the not-so-vicious-circle it has become. Of course the irony here is the body's increased need for sleep at heightened times of stress, yet inability to get it. Certainly we have all noticed a difficulty in falling asleep after a traumatic event, or even something as simple as taking on a new, uncertain project at work.

I learned a lesson during the first year I significantly increased my training volume in an effort to compete in longer races. It was the spring of 1997.

I decided to gradually increase my training mileage, about 10% per week. The first few weeks were great, no problems. Everything felt good. As the months wore on, spring became summer; I started experiencing a problem, an unexpected one. As my rate of exercise increased, my quality of sleep decreased. I found this strange. I assumed that the more exercise I did, the more tired I would be, therefore, the better I would sleep. I continued training as normal. As the weeks passed the quality of my training declined, I developed a greater appetite, and the amount of sleep I required each night increased.

I was putting my body under a great deal of physical stress. As a result, cortisol levels rose to a level that adversely affected my sleep quality. Elevated cortisol levels (dependant on severity) inhibit the body's ability to slip into the deeper, sounder sleep state known as Delta. It's in the Delta phase that the body is best able to restore itself. This is the time that regeneration takes place, facilitating improvement. Taking longer to reach Delta will obviously shorten time spent in this phase if the total sleep time remains the same. As is the case, the body needs to sleep longer to achieve the same 'restored' effect that it could have previously achieved when the level of Delta was prolonged.

To maintain the quality of my training sessions, I had to sleep an extra hour or so per night. By doing this, I got my season back on track and was able to retain my desired level of training. Though not recognizing the cause at the time, I treated the symptom, allowing myself to sleep longer. This method worked but, as I realized later, was far from optimal. Another way I could have treated the symptom would have been to reduce the amount of training performed, also far from optimal. At the time, my nutrition program was adequate, but certainly not ideal. Some of the stress I was experiencing could have been nutritionally based. Unaware of it at the time, but apparent to me now, had I nourished my overworked adrenal glands, sleep quality would have improved enough to get me back on track. If I had known about maca back then, I would have saved myself time and spared my adrenal glands the extra work.

In the years to follow, once I had learned and was able to comprehend the problem, I developed a nutrition program that would allow me to reduce the amount of uncomplementary stress placed on the body. This enabled me to maintain high levels of production stress (training), yet obtain quality Delta sleep every night. This nutrition program is the one that I outline in this book. Follow it and you will live the improvements yourself. Remember, there comes a point at which nutrition and other recovery systems are optimized, yet stress simply overwhelms them. The only way to fully recover is to reduce the amount of time you work and/or increase the amount of sleep you get. However, follow my guidelines and you can expect improved sleep quality, yielding a reduction in quantity and effectively achieving a 25-hour day.

*Lesson: Reduce stress, in particular nutritional stress, to improve sleep (which further reduces overall stress).*

## A LEAN MUSCULAR BODY - A MERE BY-PRODUCT

Training for my first Ironman triathlon, I entered into a new realm. The training was different from what I was used to, lower intensity, but much higher overall volume. Without the intense workouts, the long ones seemed much easier, for the short term. It seemed that the more volume of training I could do the better. I was putting in eight to 10 hour training days. All was well; I was becoming steadily stronger each week, as per the plan.

What began to happen next I certainly did not expect. Despite the fact that I was performing 40 hours of exercise per week, I actually began to accumulate body fat! How could this be? Was I simply eating too much, more than I could burn? Not likely. So, what was the problem? Along with being undesirable, the extra dead weight slowly being gained over the summer was decreasing my strength-to-weight ratio, certainly a reason for concern. I had to stop this from advancing any further, but how? I tried what most people would have done to lose fat, cut back on calories. After a few weeks of a calorie-reduced diet, the situation was even worse, plus now fatigue was a real concern. I remained puzzled for some time over this one.

As it turned out, the cause of this strange situation could also be attributed to the causes of the previous year's compromised sleep patterns. The answer of course was stress. Stress, primarily production (physical in this case), was what initially caused me to gain body fat. Had I trained the optimal amount, an amount that my body could recover from, I would have remained lean. As I found out later, the amount of training I was doing stressed my body to the point were my cortisol levels became chronically elevated for two months—enough to gain body fat.

My adrenal glands were exhausted, and as a result, my hormonal health sharply declined. Not aware of this at the time, I surmised that I must have simply been taking in more calories than I was burning, as is the conventional way of thinking. By reducing my caloric intake at a time when stress was already extremely high, I just exacerbated the problem. Nutritional stress had now also become a problem. Had I began to eat more instead of less I would have helped my body recover from the demands of training more efficiently. I would have actually remained leaner by eating more.

My diet then consisted primarily of carbohydrates, with a modest amount of protein and almost zero fat. A diet rich in essential fatty acids as found in whole flax and hemp foods would have provided the extra fuel that my body needed to function more efficiently, thereby reducing stress. Of course, maca would have helped bring my adrenal glands back to optimum health within weeks. Chlorella's detoxifying properties would have helped to cleanse my body, and its growth factor to speed my recovery.

An important lesson to be learned from this is that stress, even with high amounts of exercise, can cause fat to accumulate. Not eating enough nutrient-rich foods is stressful (as your body sees it). So yes, believe it or not, there are situations when eating more will reduce body fat percentage. Make sure you follow the dietary guidelines in this book, emphasizing nutrient-rich whole foods during high levels of stress.

Furthermore, if your goal is to lose body fat, be cognizant of the fact that dieting might not be the right solution. Ask yourself why it is that you have more body fat than you want. Are you overweight because you simply consume more calories than your body's activity level can utilize? If so, then yes, a reduction in total calories will help. However, if you are one of those many people who have tried a wide array of diets with marginal success, only to have the weight come back, it's time to get to the root of the problem. Follow the guidelines in this book to help you minimize nutritional stress to optimize health, that's the main requirement.

*Lesson: Consume enough nutrient-rich food to support activity level and body fat percentage will decline.*

### IMPROVE HEALTH BY MEETING NUTRITIONAL NEEDS, NOT EXCEEDING THEM

Nutritionally speaking, there are generally two types of people: those who don't care about their diet (and therefore health), and those who do. It seems that those who don't care take no supplements and those who do care take too many. 'I just want to make completely sure that I'm getting all the vitamins I need, so I take every supplement under the sun, often in large doses. My body will just excrete what it doesn't use, anyways.' While this is true of water-soluble vitamins (B and C), it is not a logical approach. However, it is a common practice, especially for athletes. Take as many supplements as you can afford to, 'just to be safe.'

As mentioned, the body does excrete the water-soluble vitamins and minerals that it doesn't need, but at what cost? It's not a high-energy cost for a healthy body to flush out unneeded vitamins, but it is still a cost. While the body is under great stress to recover from workouts the last thing you want to do is give it another job. Of course the whole reason most people take an excessive amount of supplements is in an effort to speed regeneration. Quite often they just interfere with that process, actually prolonging the time needed to complete recovery.

An excess of synthetic fat-soluble vitamins (A, D, E, K) in the system can have a considerably more severe effect than their water-soluble counterparts. Unlike water-soluble vitamins, fat-soluble vitamins remain in the system for much longer - any surplus being stored in the body's fat cells - resulting in toxicity and the symptoms that accompany it. General fatigue and weakened immune system function are the milder forms. More advanced toxicity can range from haemorrhaging to a severe reduction in intestinal flora.

Toxicity resulting from an over consumption of fat-soluble vitamins is next to impossible when whole foods are the source. The fibre contained in complete foods doesn't permit over consumption, making them the best option.

*Lesson: More vitamins are not necessarily better. A balanced approach is optimal.*

## RECALIBRATE THE BODY FOR INCREASED ENERGY

When you first get out of bed and turn on a light it seems extremely bright but is really no brighter than normal. Similarly, when sound levels are lower, the body's sense of hearing heightens. Have you ever noticed that sometimes the phone ringing sounds very loud whereas other times it sounds relatively quiet? The key word is relatively. Our body has the ability to adjust to much of what goes on around it, which serves us well. Our system automatically adapts to external stimuli; this can be good, but if misused, is to our detriment.

In order to calibrate its sensory system the body must decide at what level it will sense stimuli. The only gauge the body has is through the information we feed it: sound, sight, touch, smell, and taste. The decision will come from what 'level' we supply that information. If, for example, we drink a daily cup of coffee to increase our energy, how long does it take to notice a diminished effectiveness? Over quite a short period of time one cup of coffee will no longer have the stimulating effect on the body that it initially did. Of course the next step, as seems logical, is to drink a second cup to get the 'energy' that a single cup once delivered. Where does it end?

Our bodies are chronically over stimulated, yet most of us don't realize it – they have adapted, but at a cost. Constantly having to climb to a new level to remain in the same place is a tough way to live, yet all too common. The way to fix this problem, to help remove considerable stress from the body and thereby increase energy is to 'recalibrate' the body. Initially it will be difficult, but after about two weeks, adaptation will transpire and the results will be worth the effort. As mentioned earlier, a general improvement in diet will make the 'stripping away' of stimulants much easier, thereby allowing for recalibration.

I experimented with this theory last summer. For three days I ate nothing containing any sugar at all – including fruit. The result was a calm and productive state. At the end of the three days, I ate a few blueberries. Now, most people who have not tried this might find it strange, but by taking in just a small amount of sugar in the form of fruit had an immediate stimulating effect. I would liken it to the result formerly experienced by drinking a cup of coffee. I'm not suggesting cutting back on fruit. However, this experiment nicely underscored the value of what could be gained by recalibration.

*Lesson: Reduce stimuli to become more sensitive, resulting in easily obtainable energy through natural foods.*

## IN SPITE OF OR BECAUSE OF?

Many people subscribe to the 'If it's not broken, then don't fix it' philosophy. This thought process seems to be prevalent when it comes to diet and nutrition. This makes sense in certain situations. However, it's not a sound approach when applied to an application that has a cumulative effect. Often misunderstood, poor diet is responsible, at least in part, for many seemingly innocuous ailments. Yet, many believe that if their heart is still beating, then their diet must be okay. To a point, this is true, but I think that most people would like more from life than just survival. Again, plagued by a vicious circle, ambition and mood can be adversely affected by poor diet. Lack of motivation, and believing that you can't change or that what you want to achieve is out of reach is quite often nothing more than a sign of a chronically poor diet. How do you break the cycle? Knowledge, applied knowledge.

I know people who started eating 'health food' a few days before a race, shocked their body with the sudden change, had a bad race, and surmised, 'Health food doesn't work.' Healthy food is not a drug. Even if the change is positive, it will still take the body some time to adapt. Be patient. Gradually convert to a healthy, whole-food-based diet. Allow time for the body to adjust and your overall health can only improve. Over time, improved health will lead to improved performance.

It's true; some truly great athletes eat junk food. As many like to point out, 'look at his diet, it's full of refined, processed foods, and doesn't seem to hurt him.' These are obviously cases of an athlete being great in spite of his poor diet, not because of it.

A more extreme, yet similar point can be illustrated by a cigarette-smoking example. I could start smoking today and I could probably smoke for years, possibly decades before any clear-cut, directly related problems would arise. Naturally, there would be underlying health-related issues spanning the entire duration but they may not necessarily appear to be as symptom of smoking. It would be wrong for me to conclude that because I smoke and am okay, that smoking must not be unhealthy. We are all aware of the adverse effects of smoking. As with poor nutrition, sub-optimal performance will occur now, while the serious health problems will manifest themselves later.

Obviously, I'm an advocate of preventative methodology as opposed to the 'treat the symptom of sickness later down the road' approach. By eating nutrient-dense whole foods now, we continue to reduce chances of disease later in life and extend life expectancy.

*Lesson: Good nutrition will improve quality and quantity of life.*

## TO CARE FOR YOUR ENVIRONMENT IS TO CARE FOR YOURSELF

As a relatively new word in our language, 'environmentalist' was created to categorize a person who 'cares for his environment.' Why? Shouldn't it be self-evident that we, as human beings, take care of our surroundings? We don't have a word in our language that means 'he who cares for his family,' or 'he who values life'; these acts are the rule, not the exception.

When we bite into food, part of the environment becomes part of us. Food is our direct link; our health as a society is intimately related to the health of our food-producing earth. To not care for it, is to not care for oneself.

What can be done? Money greases the wheels of our cultural machine, therefore it is what has the greatest impact, positive or negative, on what precipitates change. This is good; we simply have to use the power of economics to help ourselves. To not support corporations that practice poor environmental policies such as unsustainable and inefficient land use, consumption of toxic pesticides and destruction of old growth forests is only half the solution. We as informed consumers hold all the power.

Many smaller, environmentally conscious companies are now beginning to grow, attracting more informed customers each year. Supporting these companies is twice as effective as just refusing to buy from ones who are destructive. For example, to buy non-genetically modified hemp foods grown without pesticides or herbicides puts money towards promoting a clean, sustainable industry. If these sustainable industries are able to flourish because of our support, others will see the economic 'carrot' of 'green agriculture,' and they will follow. This is one problem that we can eat ourselves out of!

The production, processing and delivery of food all have tremendous impact on our environment, greater than any other industry. It's pleasing to see that many people have realized the benefit organic agriculture can offer by helping to reduce the impact. However, the connection is often not made between food crops and clothing material crops. Second only to food production, and much less publicised, is the heavy chemical use of the conventional clothing industry. As with food, we can choose what kind of agriculture we support when making a clothing selection. I prefer attire made from many of the crops that also provide us some of the best food. Hemp is the strongest fibre known, resistant to mold, and able to block ultra violet rays. Linen, made from the flax plant, is strong and soft and it breathes. Experiencing a renaissance for clothing fabric, soy is exceptionally smooth and soft. Organic cotton is also excellent.

Simply by making informed decisions about what kind of agriculture we choose to support is the catalyst for change.

**Lesson: Support companies that promote environmental health.**

# Keys to creating a biologically younger, leaner body

As mentioned earlier, it is actually possible to 'grow' a younger body. A younger body is simply one that has regenerated its cells more recently. The key to maintaining (or developing) a functional, young body is to encourage it to be in a constant state of regeneration. Before the body can regenerate, it must be given a reason. That reason best comes in the form of regular exercise. Remember that exercise is really nothing more than breaking down body tissue. Its ability to grow stronger comes as a result of the regeneration process when supplied with premium fuel.

Once broken down, the body must grow new cells to replace the old. This is an ongoing process. Activity level is largely responsible for the rate at which regeneration occurs—provided of course, that the body has the resources (nutrient-rich whole foods) to support it.

*The quality of the newly-fabricated cells is solely dependant upon the fuel source supplied. When rebuilding cells, the body can go one of two ways. If it has the right resources, the new cells will be strong and healthy. However, if the only available 'building blocks' are drawn from sub-standard resources, the body has no choice but to fabricate weaker 'filler' cells. This is called degeneration, more commonly known as premature aging.*

Poor nutrition can actually convert the complementary stress that exercise provides into uncomplementary by virtue of degeneration. In fact, performing strenuous exercise regularly without eating a nutrient-rich diet will actually speed degeneration of the cells and therefore the aging process. Also, if the body is not supplied with the building blocks it needs, a stress response will be triggered, causing cortisol levels to rise and resulting in fat being stored.

How often have your heard it said, 'I did my exercise today, I'll treat myself to a cheeseburger?' Or this one: 'I've had a stressful day at work, I deserve ice cream.' People crave junk food during stressful times. Ironically, this is when it should be adamantly avoided. At the very least, make sure your body has the necessary building blocks to regenerate. Once you've seen to this, eating junk food will not be as detrimental.

*Lesson: Premium food is the key to regeneration, especially when stress is high.*

## THE HORMONE FACTOR

Hormone levels peak in the late teenage years, then begin to slowly decline. Teenagers at their peak hormone level have an easier time gaining muscle and remaining lean with little effort. As we age, one of the most significant changes that occur in our body is the gradual reduction in hormone production. As a result, we are faced with a less resilient body.

The ability to retain or regain a youthful hormonal system will yield improved immune function, the ability to gain lean muscle tissue, the reduction of body-fat percentage and an increase in vitality. Visibly reduced signs of aging, such as enhanced skin elasticity and improved agility as a result of increased tendon elasticity, are also attributes to be expected by hormonal balance.

The way to achieve balanced hormone levels is through proper nutrition as outlined in this book. A key component in the promotion of hormonal health (especially during times of augmented stress) is the regular consumption of maca. More detailed information on maca and how it works can be found on page 64.

*Lesson: Balanced hormone levels are a vital component of the anti-aging process.*

## EXERCISE

In addition to its ability to instigate regeneration, exercise has another anti-aging attribute: sweat production. Sweating helps exfoliate the pores, a necessary component of skin health. Healthy skin is more elastic and supple, giving it a youthful appearance. As mentioned earlier, a small amount of direct sun exposure is healthy. Ultraviolet rays in the sun kill bacteria that clog pores, enabling proper perspiration. Also, toxins from within the body get excreted as a component of sweat. Clear, unobstructed pours provide a vehicle for the body to maximize detoxification.

*Lesson: Exercise improves skin health and removes toxins.*

## HYDRATION

Hydration is an extremely important part of the regeneration process. When properly hydrated, the blood is thinner, enabling its efficient distribution throughout the body. Also, a hydrated body's cells swell, causing an anabolic response, therefore speeding cellular renewal. In addition, hydrated cells remain alkaline. Conversely, a catabolic response will transpire if the cells are allowed to become dehydrated, advancing degeneration.

Maintaining blood volume through proper hydration also allows:

- red blood cells to deliver oxygen to muscles efficiently
- delivery of nutrients throughout the body
- removal of waste products such as carbon dioxide
- proper hormone distribution

In addition to water, a healthy shake will also provide necessary fluid. For variety, try sipping on a nutrient rich shake throughout the morning or afternoon. As well as getting a break from water, you will be supplying your body with easily digestible health-promoting nutrition. Be aware of the fact that caffeine-containing drinks are a diuretic, and as a result, cause the body to become dehydrated.

*Lesson: Drink water throughout the day to promote regeneration.*

## FOOD BECOMES YOU - LITERALLY

We have all heard it said many times before, probably to the point that we no longer take notice, but it really is true, we are what we eat—food literally becomes us. In fact our entire body, all our muscle tissue, tendons, ligaments, skin, blood, bones, and hair did not exist a year ago as it does today. It might look similar but it is actually comprised of completely brand-new cells that have replaced the old ones. It is literally not the same body.

Your current body has been constructed from the food you've consumed over the past year. What you now biologically possess has been arrived at by four factors: diet, activity level, ability to cope with stress and genetic blueprint. How would you like your new body to look and perform? It's largely up to you. The food you eat, your activity level and how you deal with stress (three of the four determining factors) are yours for the altering. The more diligent your exercise program and the better your diet, the sooner your new body will be fabricated.

Where do our old bodies go, you ask? Most of our dead skin cells are excreted as solid waste, much is burned for energy production, some is lost in sweat; and a portion even ends up as dust in our home.

***Lesson: You CAN grow a younger body.***

## WHICH FOODS ARE BEST?

Foods rich in chlorophyll are paramount in the anti-aging process, the best sources being dark green vegetables—especially chlorella. Chlorophyll helps maintain the ever-important alkaline balance within the body and assists in the detoxification process. Providing the most concentrated form of chlorophyll, chlorella is a superfood to be eaten daily. Another unique characteristic of chlorella is its growth factor. Chlorella Growth Factor (CGF) greatly speeds the regeneration of cells, helping to quickly reconstruct body tissue. More detailed information about chlorella can be found on page 61.

Fibre is another key component. In the form of whole flax seeds, fruits, vegetables, and legumes, fibre helps control cortisol levels by stabilizing insulin while ensuring waste exits the body quickly. Having food in the body longer than necessary can cause toxins to manifest and spread.

A raw, complete protein source, such as that found in hemp, is an optimal facilitator of the regeneration process. Pea protein, also complete, provides an excellent spectrum of amino acids; complementary to that of hemp's, it yields an outstanding amino acid profile.

Maca is an anti-aging root vegetable essential for several reasons, but most notably for its ability to increase energy, assist in adaptation to stress and balance hormones naturally.

A balance of omega 3 and omega 6 essential fatty acids (EFAs), among other things, are vital for skin health. The best sources of this are hemp foods and whole flax seeds. Other raw nuts and seeds, as well as avocados, are also good. Dry skin is commonly treated topically with a moisturizer, while the cause of the problem remains un-addressed. A diet with adequate EFAs will keep skin looking and feeling supple.

As people age, their production of RNA and DNA is reduced. These two elements are essential to immune system health and cell regeneration. Healthy levels of RNA and DNA allow the body to utilize nutrients and banish toxins efficiently. As our levels drop with age, so does our ability to generate these health-promoting, anti-aging functions. To restore levels of RNA and DNA and insure that their production is constant, we need to include an adequate amount of the increasingly elusive nucleic acids in our diet. The richest source of nucleic acids in nature is chlorella.

*A recap of some excellent regenerative (anti-aging) foods:*
- **Dark leafy green vegetables**
- **Chlorella**
- **Maca**
- **Berries (especially blueberries, a very rich source of antioxidants)**
- **Hemp foods**
- **Raw nuts and seeds (especially whole flax seeds)**
- **Legumes (peas, beans and lentils)**
- **Tofu**
- **Whole grains**

If the diet is based on the foods listed above (not just supplemented with them), the body will be able to cope with 'less than ideal' foods once in a while. Anything can be eaten in moderation, however, try to avoid highly processed, refined foods. Also, anything with hydrogenated or trans fats should not be part of the diet.

**Lesson: Premium food = premium body.**

# Nutritional program outline

I have found proper nutrition to have the greatest impact on my ability to maintain a busy, full and rewarding life. The ability to curtail the debilitating attributes of stressors at the origin is invaluable. Without a cause, there can be no symptom. With no symptom, there is no need for synthetic drugs. Proper nutrition provides the mind with the clarity it needs to function optimally. It drastically speeds physical recovery from exercise and it allows the body's cells to regenerate quickly, while slowing signs of aging. Also, it helps maintain lean muscle tissue, decrease body fat, and reduces the amount of nightly sleep required, increasing productivity (or play, that's up to you) each day. To understand and harness its power is invaluable.

*Lesson: Proper nutrition will allow the body to reconstruct itself - take advantage of this.*

## ALKALINE ADVANTAGE

Alkalizing foods are an integral part of the repair process after exercise. If not dealt with, lactic acid build-up from physical exertion, general stress, or acid-forming foods will lead to muscular stiffness, fatigue, and joint pain. If an acidic system becomes chronic, it will precipitate signs of aging and will eventually cause the blood and cellular tissue to degenerate at a more rapid pace.

Daily consumption of protein with a higher pH (more alkaline) such as hemp, flax, and many other raw nuts and seeds will minimize acidity in the body. Also, a diet high in leafy green vegetables and chlorella, both excellent sources of chlorophyll, will insure the system remains alkaline. When acidic-forming food is consumed, starting with digestion and continuing through to elimination, it produces toxins that the body must deal with.

Denatured foods (those that are highly refined and processed) are devoid of any usable nutrients, yet retain their caloric value – the worst combination. Not only do denatured foods instantly create an acidic environment within the body due to their chemical composition, but they also contain toxins, leading to premature aging through cell degeneration. Aside from food, most prescription drugs, artificial sweeteners and synthetic vitamin and mineral supplements are also extremely acid forming.

As the body carries out normal functions such as movement and digestion it naturally becomes increasingly acidic. In fact, a natural by-product of healthy metabolism has an acid forming effect. This normal biological function can be taken to excess when an inordinate amount of food is consumed—another good reason to eat nutritionally-dense foods and therefore less total food.

Athletes in peak training are the most affected by excessively high acid levels (acidosis). Vigorous exercise causes lactic acid build up. Stress, of any kind, precipitates this even further. Of course physically stressed, many athletes also must deal with various types of performance anxiety. An increased metabolism is yet another factor athletes face, further lowering pH. Combine this with the fact that athletes require more food in general with an emphasis on protein to aid muscle recovery and you have all the inputs for an acid ravaged body.

Those who maintain an acidic environment within their body are also prone to fatigue. Since acidity is a stressor, cortisol levels rise resulting in impaired sleep quality.

Contrary to popular belief, it is not a lack of dietary calcium, but stress and the over-consumption of acid-forming foods and supplements that leads to most cases of poor bone health and eventually osteoporosis. The blood itself will always remain neutral; this is imperative for survival. If the body is consistently fed acid-forming, denatured foods and supplements, or encounters stress from other sources it must take measures to ensure a neutral blood pH is maintained. In doing so, the body pulls alkaline calcium from the bones. Of course over time, the bones will become weaker as a result of this survival mechanism.

The conventional way of treating low calcium levels and osteoporosis is to simply suggest the person 'take' more calcium, usually in the form of tablets. The calcium source in tablets is generally derived from materials such as oyster shells, bovine bone meal, coral and dolomite (rock), all of which are extremely hard and unnatural for the body to assimilate. Their large size and recommended daily number to be consumed is a testament to their poor bioavailability. The body must work very hard to get calcium from these sources, another reason this method of boosting calcium stores is inferior.

Low-grade metabolic acidosis as it is termed, is another symptom of an over acidic body. It has been cited as a leading cause of several health concerns such as the development of kidney stones, loss of bone mass, and the reduction of growth hormone, resulting in loss of lean muscle mass and increase of body fat production. Since low-grade metabolic acidosis affects the body at a cellular level it is also responsible for an increase in the fabrication of free radicals, and a loss in cellular energy production. In addition to these serious concerns, viral and bacterial growth is able to thrive in an acidic body, possibly leading to a wide variety of diseases. For example, it is impossible for cancer to develop in an alkaline environment; this clearly shows the importance of alkalinity in disease prevention.

Diet has the greatest impact on the body's pH level, however there are other factors to be aware of. Maintaining a positive attitude and setting time aside to do an enjoyable activity on a regular basis will further promote pH balance within the body. Taking time out of a busy schedule to do something pleasurable yet seemingly unproductive can actually be a key ingredient to improved health and longevity.

Other ways of encouraging alkalinity within the body are:

- deep breathing exercises
- yoga
- light stretching
- meditation

*Lesson: Eat foods in their natural state to help minimize acidity*

## HOW MORE PLANT-BASED FOODS CAN HELP PERFORMANCE

As you know from reading the *About the Author* section, I'm vegan, which means my diet is comprised solely of plant-based foods. When implemented properly, I believe a vegan diet is an optimal one for performance. However, even if a strict animal-free diet is not for you, principles from it can complement an existing eating plan with impressive results.

First, I choose a daily dose of a complete, raw plant protein. Raw plant protein is superior for several reasons. Naturally occurring live enzymes, present only in raw protein, are absorbed and utilized in a far more efficient manner than processed proteins. Feeding the body natural whole food sources of protein greatly reduces the amount needed by improving efficacy. Furthermore, raw plant protein has a higher pH than many 'manufactured' sources such as whey protein and other isolates. As you know from the alkaline advantage section of this book, it really is an advantage. Raw hemp protein is my first choice. It's also extremely high in naturally occurring vitamin E, a powerful antioxidant.

Dark leafy green vegetables are a rich source of chlorophyll, important in the reduction of lactic acid, a destructive by-product of exercise. Chlorophyll also cleanses and oxygenates the blood, making it an essential 'modern world' food and a true performance enhancer. More available oxygen in the blood translates to better endurance and an overall reduction in fatigue. In their raw state, chlorophyll-containing plants possess an abundance of live enzymes that promote the quick rejuvenation of our cells. The consumption of chlorophyll-rich, raw plant food combined with moderate exercise is the best way to create a biologically younger body. My favourite green food is chlorella because it is the richest source of chlorophyll and nucleic acids in nature, plus it provides a reliable supply of vitamin B12.

Maca, aside from its myriad of nutrients (trace amounts of 31 minerals) can supply the body with a non-stimulating form of energy. Maca's ability to deliver energy is by means of hormonal regulation and adrenal nourishment, not stimulation. As the diet improves, maca's energy-inducing properties become increasingly apparent.

The digestive ease and bioavailability of most plant foods also contribute advantages. Fatigue, bloating, cramping, and an upset stomach can often be attributed to poor digestion. Many whole plant foods (especially those rich in chlorophyll) have enzymes intact to accommodate quick and efficient digestion. The quicker nutrients can be extracted from food, the sooner it can be eliminated, which is a key factor for optimal health. Also, insoluble fibre-containing plant matter further speeds waste through the system, reducing the risk of toxic manifestation, starting in the colon and spreading throughout.

## HELP YOUR BODY HELP YOU - HAVE A NUTRITIOUS SHAKE DAILY

Traditionally, drinking a nutrient-packed shake on a daily basis was relegated to athletes and dieters. However, there are benefits for all. Shakes are becoming more popular with people from all walks of life for several reasons.

It's easy to pack nutrients into liquid form thereby improving assimilation; basically allowing the body to get what it wants while expending less energy to get it. I have one or more nutrient-packed shakes daily to insure that I get all the nutrients I need to support my activity level and induce a quick recovery.

*Consuming an easily assimilated meal in liquid form gives the digestive system a break, further reducing overall stress. A daily liquid meal allows for better recovery because not as much blood is needed in the stomach to process it. Blood can remain 'working' in the extremities, delivering nutrients and oxygen, removing waste products produced by exercise and other stresses, speeding the alkaline balance and advancing recovery.*

Also, since it's important to eat several meals and/or snacks a day, it's convenient to make one or more of the liquid variety when you're busy.

## WHAT A NUTRITIOUS SHAKE SHOULD CONTAIN

Ideally, a shake should contain all the nutrients that a complete meal does. First, make sure that the protein is of an easily digestible source. Otherwise, one of the health promoting benefits a shake offers ease of digestibility will be reduced. The protein is best obtained from whole food that has as high a pH as possible and at least a portion of it should be derived from a raw source, such as hemp. Raw hemp protein is packed with live enzymes that improve digestion and absorption. Hemp is unique in its ability to provide a high amount of complete protein in raw form, which I have found to be most valuable. I always use hemp protein as my primary protein source when making a shake.

For high quality fat, such as omega-3, I use ground-up whole flax seeds. Flax also provides soluble fibre and a small amount of complete protein. Maca, as an adaptogen, adrenal tonic and a source of sterols and sterolins, is also a critical ingredient. Chlorella, for its detoxifying properties, naturally occurring vitamin B12, growth factor, nucleic acids and rich chlorophyll content, make it a worthy addition. Chlorella is also an excellent source of complete raw protein (65%). Hemp, flax, maca and chlorella are the four primary shake ingredients. After adding them, I fill it up with fruit (whole, not juice). Berries are always desirable as they are loaded with antioxidants. One of my favourite shake recipes is on page 87. Feel free to experiment with all kinds of fruit for variety. Raw carob powder is also a nice addition.

In an attempt to optimize the nutritional value of this recipe I began adding pea and rice protein powder to balance the amino acid profile. I also, started adding pre and probiotics, enzymes and a concentrated berry complex. As you can imagine the daily creation of this shake became cumbersome and time consuming, spurring me on to create Vega. For the complete story behind Vega's creation please see page 94.

## TIMING OF NUTRITION

A commonly applied weight-loss strategy practiced by some is to restrict calorie intake immediately following a workout. I know many people who will go for a long run, then not eat for several hours after, in an attempt to shed body fat. These are the same people who wonder why they feel lethargic during their next workout, and eventually need to skip workouts to feel 'rejuvenated.' In addition to missed workouts, other signs of stress become evident within a couple of weeks. Cortisol levels rise, actually causing the body to retain body fat and cannibalize muscle tissue, which is certainly not the desired effect.

Immediately following a workout, a snack comprised of primarily sugary, starchy foods should be eaten. If you have a sweet tooth, within 45 minutes following a workout is when you can exercise it. The post-workout snack is unique. To speed recovery, the body needs sugar to enter the bloodstream as fast as possible. Therefore, this snack should contain very little fat (even the good kind), and no fibre. A small amount of protein is okay, but no more than 25% of the total snack.

My 'recovery pudding' on page 80 contains the correct ratio: the banana and pear provide both simple and complex carbohydrates as well as electrolytes lost in sweat. The tofu supplies a small amount of protein, just enough to assist the carbohydrate in the muscle glycogen regeneration processes. A small amount of hemp oil helps to advance the repair of soft tissue damage, an inevitable by-product of exercise. These foods, especially once blended together, are very easy for the fatigued body to digest and utilize.

After an hour has passed since your post-exercise snack, it's time for a complete, nutrient-rich meal. Ideally, this meal is best comprised of high-quality, easily-digestible raw protein such as hemp, omega-3 fatty acids (also from hemp and flax), and a full spectrum of vitamins and minerals. A nutritious shake can be a convenient and effective solution as long as it is complete.

Timing of nutrition is an often over-looked aspect of overall health. It is possible to eat all the right food but at less than optimal times, therefore inhibiting effectiveness. For example, a snack high in dense carbohydrate is an ideal one to boost muscle glycogen levels and speed recovery following a training session. Yet, it would inhibit the release of growth hormone if consumed close to bedtime. A high protein meal a few hours after exercise can help aid in the repair of muscle tissue. Conversely, a high protein meal immediately following exercise can inhibit proper hydration, leading to prolonged recovery. A sugary snack during an intense training session can improve endurance by supplying the muscles with readily-available fuel, whereas a sugary snack eaten while sitting in front of a computer will, within an hour or so, make concentration harder and precipitate fatigue.

## MAXIMIZE RECOVERY BEFORE THE WORKOUT EVEN BEGINS

My goal is to ensure that my body is properly fuelled at all times so that what is consumed immediately before a workout is insignificant. If the body must have nourishment before a workout to perform properly, it's a sign that its requirements have not been met earlier. That being said, sometimes it is useful to consume a small pre-workout snack for insurance purposes, especially prior to long training sessions. Being adequately hydrated and fuelled before exercise begins, in addition to maintaining it throughout, will decrease the amount of stress placed on the body, therefore aid recovery.

The key requirement for a pre-workout snack is ease of digestibility. Before short workouts I'll usually just have a banana. However, if I'm going to perform a particularly long or intense session I'll make Vega energy pudding, recipe on page 89. It digests very quickly and supplies the nutrients required to sustain high-level performance for an extended period, increasing time between refuelling.

One objective that I set for myself during exercise is to never get thirsty or hungry. Knowing that I'll feel the first onset of thirst at about the 20-minute mark, I'll be sure to drink 15 minutes in. During workouts projected to last longer than 90 minutes, but under two hours, I'll have a sip of water every 15 minutes. I apply the same philosophy to eating while training. For exercise sessions exceeding 2 hours, I'll be sure to consume some easily digestible nutrients as well, about every 25 minutes. For this, I developed the Vega sport drink, recipe on page 88 and the Vega energybar, recipe on page 91.

Within 45 minutes of completing a workout it's ideal to consume some easily digestible foods such as my recovery pudding on page 80. Easily digestible fruit such as bananas, mangos and papayas are also an excellent option upon completing a longer workout. I let the fruit digest for about 30 minutes then consume a liquid whole meal such as a Vega shake. In doing so, my body will get all the nutrients in a pH balanced, liquid form that is easily digestible and absorbable.

Consuming a liquid meal is of increased value shortly after exercise because the majority of the blood will be busy, rapidly circulating throughout the body, clearing lactic acid and other metabolic waste from the extremities and delivering nutrients. The consumption of a traditional meal at this time will require a large amount of blood to travel to the stomach to aid in the digestion process. Of course since the blood is needed in the stomach it cannot remain in the extremities going about its 'clean up and delivery' job. With the extra strain of digestion removed by consuming complete liquid nutrition, recovery will dramatically improve.

**Lesson: Reduce the importance of a pre-workout snack by laying the groundwork for recovery before the workout begins.**

# Favourite foods

My eating plan is structured around whole foods, not merely supplemented with them. The following are my favourite foods; ones I eat consistently, comprising an integral part of my diet. I choose non-genetically modified, organic versions whenever possible.

## CHLORELLA: THE ULTIMATE GREEN FOOD

One of the finest superfoods in nature is chlorella, a single-celled freshwater microscopic green algae. I could write a whole book just on chlorella's amazing attributes and practical applications. Capable of reproducing itself four times every 24 hours, chlorella is the fastest growing plant on earth. It also contains more chlorophyll, DNA and RNA than any other plant. With all these accolades, it's no surprise that chlorella is the number one supplement in Japan with over 10 million regular users.

Popularized out of necessity in Japan due to a scarcity of land, chlorella is being investigated by the west as a 'land saver.' Its amazing rate of growth has made it a subject of study for scientists who aim to improve food-producing land yields. Chlorella is 65% protein, making it by far the most environmentally efficient method of protein production. Contrast this to whey protein where grazing land is needed for the cattle and farm land is needed to grow grains to feed the cows. The cows have to then be milked, the whey extracted, then the protein extracted from the whey etc.—all a draw on resources. Plus, since chlorella has the highest level of chlorophyll of any organism, the protein remains alkaline, thus speeding recovery.

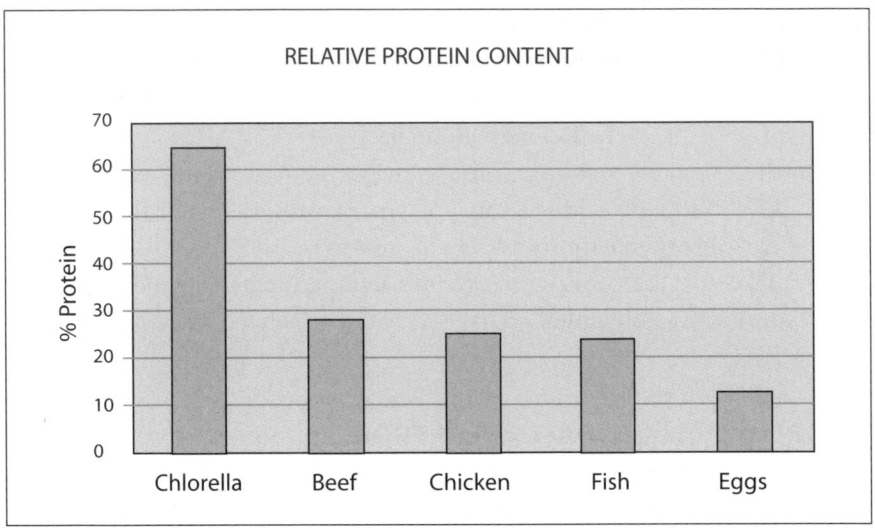

Chlorella is a complete food; it can also be considered a vitamin and mineral supplement. Nutritionally speaking, chlorella is a true super-food, containing 65% protein, essential fatty acids, and a plethora of vitamins, minerals and enzymes. Also, chlorella contains the elusive (at least, in the plant kingdom) vitamin B12, which is extremely hard for vegetarians to find in forms other than laboratory-created tablets. Chlorella provides it, naturally.

Chlorella possesses 19 different amino acids. Among them are all 10 of the essential ones. Essential amino acids are ones that must be obtained through diet. The body cannot manufacture them; therefore chlorella is a complete protein. The amino acids present, in conjunction with naturally occurring enzymes, are the most easily absorbed and utilized form of protein available. The ease at which these amino acids can be utilized is yet another 'task' removed from the body. Many other complete proteins are much more 'energy intensive' to digest.

So complete is this wonder-food that, when consuming nothing other than chlorella, human life can be sustained for an extended period of time. This was discovered by NASA when the space agency was looking at ways to sustain astronauts for extended space travel.

Another key component, its detoxification properties, has recently garnered chlorella some attention in the west. As we know all too well, our air and water quality is getting worse. There really is no practical way to avoid our exposure to it. I choose chlorella as a daily body detoxifier. It helps reduce stress on the system from environmental pollutants. At times, I have no choice but to ride my bike on streets with heavy traffic, en route to more suitable training grounds, so I must still pass through polluted air. Chlorella aids in the reduction in cellular damage incurred by free radicals, produced by vehicle emissions.

When consumed daily, chlorella is a perfect example of a preventative measure taken to build better health via a stronger body. Directly enhancing the immune system at a cellular level, chlorella treats the cause of any possible breach, as opposed to fighting the onset of sickness (as is all too often done with pharmaceutical drugs).

Nucleic acids (RNA and DNA) and Chlorella Growth Factor (CGF), a compound exclusively found in chlorella, are attributes that set it apart. CGF is what is responsible for chlorella's unprecedented ability to quadruple everyday. By consuming chlorella, we can benefit from its growth factor. It speeds cell regeneration, slows signs of aging, enhances healing and expedites muscle recovery. Important to note, CGF is capable of stimulating tissue repair even when the body's healing sources are overworked due to incessant stress. The CGF is capable of swinging immune function north of the proverbial 'fine line' during time of unrelenting stress, thus avoiding sickness.

When selecting chlorella, be sure to look for one with a high level of CGF. The amount of CGF is what differentiates various types of chlorella, so select the highest possible. Also important is to look for high levels of protein and chlorophyll. These three factors are the most important ones to consider when choosing a brand of chlorella.

Since chlorella is a whole food, a daily dose of at least 1.5 grams is recommended, 2.5 grams daily is significantly better. Personally, I consume up to

7.5 grams (1 tbsp) a day during heavy training, resulting in notable performance improvement.

## MACA: ADAPTOGEN AND HORMONAL BALANCER

Maca is another favourite food of mine. A root vegetable from the Peruvian highlands, grown in mineral-rich volcanic soil, maca is another true superfood. Used as a staple by native Peruvians for thousands of years, maca allowed them to prosper in the high mountain regions they inhabit.

Maca is known as an adaptogen. When the Spanish conquistadors invaded Peru, they had tremendous trouble adapting to their new environment. Accustomed to sea level, the newcomers now had to adapt to the new land that lay at 11,000 to 15,000 feet in elevation. At this altitude, oxygen in the air is less than half of what it is at sea level. Physically stressed beyond their limits, the newcomers were having great difficulty. Their livestock, also new to the region, were clearly exhibiting signs of stress as well. Their fatigue became evident and their fertility declined. Fed maca, the animals soon adapted to the debilitating stress their harsh new environment had thrust upon them. Making the connection, the conquistadors began eating maca also with similar results.

Curtailing the effects of stress by aiding the regeneration of the adrenal glands, maca is an ideal 'modern world' food. Personally, I have found a greater ability to adapt to physical stress when supplementing with maca. Also, due to the negative effect that stress has on hormonal health, maca works to restore it. Even a modest decline—or increase, for that matter— in certain hormone levels will impair the ability to build muscle and recover from stress in general. An out-of-balance hormonal system is a catalyst for numerous ailments. In addition to sickness, a prolonged hormonal imbalance will induce signs of premature aging and cause excess body fat to be stored.

As mentioned earlier in this book, balance is the key to either adapting to physical stress, therefore becoming stronger, or having it overwhelm your system. I've found with maca that I'm able to continue training at a high level while maintaining hormone balance, thereby prolonging the amount I can train and adapt to.

Maca also possesses the building blocks or precursors for the production of serotonin. As mentioned earlier, the body will quite often try to 'self-medicate' when it's feeling overwhelmed by stress-induced chemical reactions in the brain. It's at this time that sugar cravings are often prevalent, in the brain's attempt to raise serotonin levels. However, a diet that includes a daily dose of maca will supply the body with what it needs to curtail stress and construct serotonin, thereby reducing or altogether eliminating sugar cravings and the vicious circle they can induce.

Sterols are steroid-like compounds found in both plants and animals. Maca is a rich source of sterols, which promote quick regeneration of fatigued muscle tissue. As mentioned earlier, phasing of training is vital for optimal results. During the off-season, I make a concerted effort to build strength and muscle mass in the gym. Strength is important for any athlete, even an endurance athlete. It improves the efficiency of muscle contractions. I also like to start the season with a bit more muscle than I need since it will be whittled down as the year progresses. I've recently experienced exceptional strength gains while supplementing with maca. I've had the ability to lift more weight than in previous years and in addition, the ability to recover faster. It has enabled me to perform more high quality workouts, thereby advancing my progress. Also, important to note, maca increases energy by means of nourishment, not stimulation.

When selecting maca, be sure to choose the gelatinized form for best results. Gelatinization is a process that removes the hard-to-digest starchy component of the maca root. The result is an easily-digestible, quickly assimilated and more concentrated form of maca. Gelatinized maca has a pleasant, nutty taste and dissolves more easily than regular maca. Most importantly, the published human clinical studies proving maca's effectiveness were all performed using the gelatinized form.

As with chlorella, I suggest at least 1.5 grams daily, 2.5 is better. Also, as with chlorella, I personally consume much more during times of heavy training; up to 7.5 grams (1 tbsp) daily, with excellent results.

## HEMP: THE FINEST SOURCE OF RAW PROTEIN IN NATURE

Hemp foods have been gaining popularity over the past few years, and for good reason. Hemp has many qualities that set it apart from most other foods, attributes especially important for athletes and active and/or busy people. First, hemp is a nutrient-rich whole food in its natural state. There's no need to create isolates or extracts from it. As you know from the *Alkaline advantage* section, hemp in its whole-food state has a higher pH than many other proteins, which is of utmost importance, yet commonly overlooked by many when selecting a protein source.

The protein present in hemp is complete, containing all 10 essential amino acids. When included in the diet, the full spectrum of essential amino acids, possessed by hemp, becomes a clear advantage to any active individual. Hemp's amino acid profile will facilitate a boost in the immune system and hasten recovery, making it superior to other sources of protein. Hemp foods also have natural anti-inflammatory properties, key factors for speeding the repair of soft tissue damage caused by physical activity. Edestin, an amino acid present primerly in hemp, is considered an integral part of DNA. It makes hemp the closest plant source to our own human amino acid profile.

I find the digestibility of hemp protein to be superior to all others I've tried. Since hemp protein is raw, its naturally occurring digestive enzymes remain intact, allowing it to be used by the body with the greatest of ease.

Superior digestibility and relatively high pH of hemp make it possible for the body to utilize it better, therefore reducing the body's protein requirements. As a result, the digestive strain placed on the body to absorb and utilize protein is reduced. Quality, not quantity is paramount. Also, because hemp foods are raw, they maintain their naturally high level of vitamins, minerals, high-quality balanced fats, antioxidants, fibre and the very alkaline chlorophyll.

High-quality complete protein such as hemp is an instrumental part of not only muscle tissue regeneration, but also fat metabolism. Protein ingestion instigates the release of a hormone that enables the body to more easily utilize its fat reserves, thereby improving endurance and facilitating body fat loss.

Along with being nutritionally superior, hemp is also environmentally superior. Unlike many crops, hemp can be grown in both hot and cold environments, making use of land that could not possibly produce as high a yield with another crop. Growing much faster than many crops, hemp can be harvested in less time, allowing more to be produced. Naturally resistant to most pests, hemp crops can be grown efficiently without the use of herbicides or pesticides.

Hemp crops have actually been planted in over-farmed fields to 'rejuvenate' the soil. Once the hemp has grown its cycle, it gets ploughed into the soil to decompose. After a few rotations, the land can then be used for the production of 'less versatile' crops. Hemp can thrive in arid conditions, making irrigation unnecessary, thereby conserving water. Since much of the water used to irrigate crops is far from pure, hemp becomes exempt from the possible health concerns impure water can impose. The health of our environment is directly related to our health as a society. Choosing to support sustainable agriculture is to choose a cleaner environment and a healthier society.

Freshness is particularly important when selecting hemp foods. A deep, rich green colour, pleasant smell and sweet, nutty taste are indications of a recent harvest. As with any crop, be sure to choose hemp that has been grown without the use of herbicides and pesticides.

## FLAX: GREATEST OMEGA-3 SOURCE IN THE PLANT KINGDOM

Out of the entire plant kingdom, flax contains the highest level of omega-3, an essential fatty acid. Omega-3 and omega-6 are considered essential because, like essential amino acids, the body cannot produce them. Omega 6 is relatively easy to obtain in a healthy diet; it is prevalent in many nuts, seeds and vegetable oils. In contrast, omega-3 is relatively rare in the plant kingdom, although hemp and walnuts contain some. Flax, however, is the most abundant source of omega-3 (57 per cent of total fat), making it a vital addition to the vegetarian or vegan diet.

Omega-3 is of major importance for the athlete. Aside from its ability to help reduce inflammation caused by movement, omega-3 plays an integral part in the metabolism of fat. A diet with a daily dose of 10 grams (about 1 tablespoon) of whole flax seeds will allow the body to more efficiently burn body fat as fuel. This is obviously a beneficial attribute to anyone wanting to shed body fat, but it is of major importance to athletes who need to spare muscle glycogen. As the body becomes proficient at burning fat as fuel (by training and proper diet), endurance significantly improves.

Let's compare two athletes, both with an equal level of fitness. One relies purely on his body's ability to burn carbohydrates, while the other has fueled his body with high-quality fats as well. The purely carbohydrate-fed athlete's muscles can only store enough muscle glycogen for about a 90 minute workout. After that, more needs to be ingested or performance will decline. Conversely, the athlete who has incorporated omega-3 and omega-6 in his diet (and trained properly) will have the ability to draw from his fat reserves. This is significant because, he then has a dual fuel source. This will prolong the amount of time it takes for his muscle glycogen to be depleted, while improving endurance—not to mention creating a leaner body.

Whole flax seeds are high in potassium, an integral electrolyte for active people, which is responsible in part for smooth muscle contractions. Potassium is lost in sweat so it must be replaced regularly to keep serum levels adequately stocked. Potassium also helps to maintain fluid balance, assisting with the hydration process.

Flax also contains both soluble and insoluble fibre. Soluble fibre slows the release of carbohydrates into the bloodstream, helping to control insulin levels and prolong energy. Also, soluble fibre gives the body a sense of fullness, signaling its hunger mechanism to shut off. For this reason, people who are trying to lose weight are advised to increase their consumption of soluble fibre. Insoluble fibre is important in terms of digestive system health. Insuring toxins don't build up and spread to the bloodstream, insoluble fibre plays a cleansing role.

Like hemp, flax also has anti-inflammatory properties, a welcome addition to any active person's life. Also a whole food, and a complete protein with all essential amino acids present, flax retains its enzymes, allowing it to be absorbed and utilized by the body with ease, improving immune function.

Be sure to select whole flax seed, not flax seed meal. Whole flax seeds contain all their health promoting oils, nutrients, enzymes, vitamins and minerals. Flax meal is what is left over after the oils have been extracted from the whole flax seed. Nutritionally speaking, flax meal is mostly fibre and is commonly used as filler in baked goods or low-end meal replacements. I suggest buying whole flax seeds, grinding them in a coffee grinder, and then storing them in the fridge.

## LEGUMES: GREAT SOURCE OF PROTEIN AND FIBRE

Legumes are a variety of plant that has pods with small seeds inside. They include lentils, peas, beans, and peanuts. Lentils and split peas are among the most commonly used legumes for the simple reason that they don't need to be soaked before cooking. In about as much time as it takes to cook pasta, lentils and split peas can be prepared.

Legumes in general have an excellent nutritional profile. High in protein, fibre, and many vitamins and minerals, a variety of legumes are part of my regular diet. Peas, in particular yellow, have an exceptional amino acid profile. Also rich in B vitamins (responsible in part for converting food into energy) and potassium (an electrolyte needed for smooth muscle contractions), yellow peas are an excellent addition to an active person's diet. Due to the superior amino acid profile in peas, several manufacturers are now producing pea protein concentrates and isolates. A good option for a high quality vegetarian protein source, pea protein is also beneficial for those with soy allergies.

Avoided by some because of their gas producing reputation, legumes are actually no more a culprit than many other foods, as long as they are prepared properly. After soaking beans and shelled peas in preparation for cooking, be sure to rinse them in fresh water. Also, rinse them in fresh water after they have been cooked. The water they soak and cook in will absorb some of the indigestible sugars that cause gas; rinsing it off will help improve digestion and minimize gas production. As with all fibre rich foods, legumes should be introduced slowly into the diet, so to allow time for the digestion system to adapt. Progressively increasing the amount of legumes eaten will ensure a smooth transition to a healthier diet.

Sprouting various types of legumes is another preparation method. Sprouting improves both the nutritional value and digestibility; enabling the legumes to be consumed raw. Sprouting also allows the digestive enzymes to remain intact, eliminating gas production altogether.

## SOY PROTEIN: CONVENIENT SOURCE OF PROTEIN

Soy is available in several powdered forms, among the most common are flour, fermented and isolate. Soy flour has a 1:1 ratio of protein to carbohydrate, making it a good substitute for many starchier flours when used in baking. Fermented soy is most commonly used as an alterative for people who have difficulty digesting complete soy foods. The fermentation process utilizes probiotic bacteria to start the digestion process even before you put it in your mouth.

Isolate is the most commonly used form of soy protein, simply because of its extremely high protein content (over 90%). As the name suggests, the protein has been isolated from the rest of the soybean. For a quick, convenient protein hit, isolate is good. However, keep in mind that due to its processing, it is no longer a whole food. Also, it is acidic; therefore, I suggest only eating soy protein isolate with alkalizing foods such as dark leafy green vegetables. For a full-spectrum, complete protein alternative, try pea protein - it also has an excellent amino acid profile.

## TOFU: HIGH QUALITY, VERSATILE PROTEIN

Tofu is another high-quality complete protein made from soy. Easy to digest, tofu is a good choice for active people. The versatility of tofu has made it part of the mainstream North American food culture. As an ideal transition food for those making an effort to cut down on their consumption of meat, tofu has served its purpose well. Try to choose tofu made from non-genetically modified, organic soybeans.

## WHOLE GRAINS: HIGH QUALITY CARBOHYDRATE

When most people think of whole grains, they think of whole wheat. While there's nothing wrong with whole wheat, unless you have a sensitivity to gluten, there are many other grains available to add variety to a healthy diet.

Whole grains, as the name suggests, means nothing has been extracted. A large number of the grain products currently in our food chain have been refined. Most bread, pizza crust, and other conventional baked-goods are made with refined, or what is also referred to as, processed flour. Refined flours have had their fibre and protein removed, and as a result most of the vitamins and minerals have also been extracted. All that remains is a nutrient-absent starch. The reason for the extensive use of nutrient-absent flour is primarily cost related. Also, refined flour will be lighter, therefore allowing it to rise more and be 'fluffier', which has become desirable. The problem is; not only does refined flour not provide us with the nutrients we need to function optimally, it also causes insulin levels to sharply rise, inducing a stress response and weight gain. When in their natural, unadulterated state, grain products provide an excellent steady stream of lasting energy.

Also worth mentioning, some grains are more alkaline than others. Those with the highest pH should be consumed more frequently, while the others, eaten in moderation. Grains to be eaten most often because they are gluten free and alkaline are amaranth, quinoa, millet, wild rice, brown rice and buckwheat (not actually wheat - contains no gluten). More acidic, but still good, grains include whole wheat, spelt and kamut. When selecting grain products, be sure to choose organic and non-genetically modified.

## SESAME SEEDS: RICH IN CALCIUM

Sesame seeds are an excellent, easily absorbable source of calcium. In part, calcium is responsible for muscle contractions, making its correct serum level important for athletes. It is also important in the formation and maintenance of bones and teeth. Excreted in sweat, more dietary calcium is needed in the diets of athletes and those individuals living in a warm climate.

I grind sesame seeds into a flour in a coffee grinder, keep it in the fridge and sprinkle it on salads, cereal, pasta, soups, and anything else I can think of. I also use this sesame seed flour in many of my recipes to enhance calcium content. When baking, try substituting some of the regular flour with sesame seed flour.

## PUMPKIN SEEDS: GREAT SOURCE OF IRON

Pumpkin seeds are iron-rich. Iron is another nutrient some people have trouble getting enough of, especially those who don't eat meat. Anemia is a concern for some. Apart from low dietary iron, anemia can be precipitated by strenuous exercises. Iron is lost as a result of compression hemolysis (crushed blood cells due to intense muscle contractions). The more active the person, the more dietary iron is needed.

Constant impact activity, such as running, reduces iron levels more dramatically due to a more strenuous form of hemolysis. With each foot strike, a small amount of blood is released from the damaged capillaries. In time, this will cause anemia if close attention to diet is not paid. Iron is also lost through sweat. I always keep raw pumpkin seeds on hand, sprinkling them on a wide variety of foods.

## GINGER: ANTI-INFLAMMATORY ASSISTANT

Fresh, whole ginger is a worthy addition to any diet. Ginger can help the digestion process and ease an upset stomach. Personally, I use it raw in many recipes. Ginger has anti-inflammatory properties, therefore can aid in the recovery of soft tissue injuries and help promote quicker healing of strains. I load up on ginger as my mileage increases to insure inflammation is kept under control. Any food with anti-inflammatory properties is of value since inflammation hastens signs of aging.

## Enzymes: Essential for proper digestion

Enzymes are one of the least appreciated yet most important components of our diet. An absence of enzymes can result in the same sickness and disease associated with malnutrition, even if a perfect diet is adhered to. Without enzymes, food cannot be turned into usable fuel for the body. As with hormonal level, enzyme production diminishes with age, leaving us solely reliant on diet.

In the distant past, that was of little concern, as enzymes were plentiful in food. Once relatively easy to obtain, enzyme profusion is declining, while our sickness increases. Coincidence? Probably not. Poor dietary habits and stress are again the root of the problem. As our fresh whole food choices dwindle, making way for highly refined, processed 'shells' of their former incarnation, we now lack enzymes in our food. In addition to the diminishing enzyme level in food, poor diet further depletes the system. The digestion process of starchy, sugary and fatty foods is a major draw on body-produced enzymes, further diminishing its precious supply.

In addition to dietary shortcomings, enzymes are destroyed by stress. Nutritional stress damages cells that enzymes are in part required to reconstruct. Stress also inhibits the body's ability to produce enzymes, another vicious circle. Pollutants in the air are a draw on the immune system and again enzymes are called upon to fortify it.

The speed and quality of cell reconstruction after exercise is partly dependant on enzyme prevalence. Without enough, the whole process will slow, speeding signs of aging. Again, the vicious circle is created. Low enzymatic levels, formed in part by stress, slow the repair of stress-related damage, precipitating the problem.

Raw food still has enzymes intact, but only enough to help it to be properly digested. Eating more raw foods is certainly a good way to get more enzymes in the diet. However, cooked foods are completely void of enzymes, therefore making supplementation a good option.

Enzymatically speaking, the ideal situation would be for all of us to eat only raw, organic food the day that it's harvested, not be exposed to any form of environmental pollutants, and live a stress-free life. Obviously, this is not realistic in our modern world.

Consuming a daily dose of raw foods, reducing uncomplementary stress (mostly through proper nutrition), avoiding enzyme-depleting foods (starchy, deep-fried) is a step in the right direction. For optimal health and performance, consider supplementing with natural enzymes.

## PROBIOTICS: FRIENDLY INTESTINAL FLORA

Probiotic is a Greek word, which means 'for life.' Known as 'good' bacteria, probiotics support beneficial intestinal flora. A positive balance of good intestinal flora will help the body digest, process and utilize complex carbohydrates and protein. Also, the regular consumption of probiotics increases the bioavailability of minerals, especially calcium.

As mentioned in an earlier chapter, if nutrient-rich whole foods are not primary, cravings and over-eating will develop. If they persist, even though you are adhering to a nutrient-rich diet, the problem could be absorption. Once food has been digested in the stomach, it's free to leave. However it still has a few responsibilities. First, it passes into the intestine, where the vitamins and minerals are absorbed for utilization. If good bacteria is not prevalent in the intestine, the absorption process will be hindered. Not being able to utilize vitamin-rich foods is just as bad as not consuming them in the first place.

As a society, we know all too well that when we get a bacterial infection, we are given antibiotics to kill it. The problem with this is that antibiotics also kill good bacteria. Increasingly, antibiotics don't work as well as they have in the past, as many bacteria have developed resistance to them. Again, it's about prevention. By ensuring probiotics are consumed daily, the chance of infection—and therefore the need for antibiotics—is greatly reduced. Consistent probiotic use has shown to dramatically improve immune function. I personally take 250mg of dairy-free probiotics daily.

## Stevia: Sweet blood sugar regulator

Stevia is classified as an herb, native to Paraguay. The intense sweetness of its leaf is stevia's most celebrated feature. About 30 times sweeter than sugar, dried stevia leaf contains no carbohydrates and therefore has zero effect on insulin levels. Stevia has actually shown to help equalize blood sugar levels raised by other sugars and starch consumed at the same time. Stevia, as you might expect, is quickly gaining popularity among those in pursuit of a leaner body for use as a natural sugar substitute. A much better alternative to laboratory-created artificial sweeteners, stevia leaf is a whole food, just dried and ground into powder.

I personally use stevia as an additive to many of my foods. Its ability to help regulate blood sugar levels is important for sustained energy. It improves the energy release of food it's eaten with. I even add stevia to my sport drink to help improve its effectiveness. Improved digestion is another benefit of stevia.

## Sprouts: Nutrient packed

Not quite a plant yet no longer a seed, the sprout occupies a special transitional phase in the plant life cycle. Having yet to form roots, the sprout cannot feed itself, and therefore must rely on the nutrients contained within its seed. Once activated by moisture, enzymes begin to utilize nutrients supplied in the seed as a rapid growth fuel. The plant equivalent of mother's milk, densely packed nutrients quickly convert the sprout into a plant.

Of great interest to many grazing animals and us humans alike, the sprout has much to offer. Throughout this rapid growth phase, digestive enzyme inhibitors are expelled, proteins are converted to amino acids and fats into essential fatty acids, and a form of pre-digestion occurs, making for a very efficient food. Power-packed with vitamins, minerals, chlorophyll and enzymes, sprouts greatly enhance the efficiency and nutrient value of the seed. Possessing a high pH level, sprouts will also help alkalize the body.

Sprouting works for most grains, legumes, nuts and seeds. Though not technically considered sprouts, since they don't produce a shoot, soaking raw nuts and seeds overnight will still provide all the same benefits. Almonds, pumpkin seeds and sesame seeds are the ones I soak most often. Quinoa, often referred to as a grain but technically a seed, is also ideal for sprouting thereby unleashing its full array of nutrients.

After soaking or sprouting, be sure to rinse the sprouts in fresh water. This will wash off the digestive inhibiters that have leached into the water, thus improving bioavailability.

## SEA VEGETABLES: NATURAL ELECTROLYTE CONCENTRATE

Generally referred to as seaweed, dulse, nori, and kelp are the best-known sea vegetables to North Americans. Seaweed, also referred to as wild ocean plant, is an exceptionally good source of minerals and trace elements. Dulse, for example, provides the perfect mineral complex in a natural form. The daily consumption of natural-source minerals and trace elements is important for optimal health. Especially significant for active people, adequate mineral consumption allows the cells to stay hydrated longer, thereby improving endurance. Sea vegetables are a superior source, since they are also chlorophyll-rich and alkaline-forming.

## Yerba maté: Nutrient rich leaf

Yerba maté is a South American plant most commonly used for making an infused tea-like drink from the leaf. Similar to green tea in many respects, yerba maté poseses several numeros health-promoting properties. Rich in chlorophyll, antioxidants and numerous trace minerals, yerba maté is also a good digestive aid. For these reasons, I use it in several of my recipes.

Yerba maté is mostly grown in Paraguay. When selecting yerba maté, be sure to choose one that is either 'wild harvest' or has been grown 'with' the jungle, not instead of the jungle. Avoid 'plantation style' farms that have cleared old-growth forest. Supporting farmers of wild harvest yerba maté, it enables them to economically prosper, making the need to clear old-growth rain forest unnecessary. As long as their product is economically viable to produce, the land will not be cleared for the farming of animals.

## Dates: Premium quick fuel

High in the carbohydrate glucose, dates are sometimes referred to as 'Nature's Fuel.' Upon consumption, glucose is rapidly converted to glycogen in the liver. Maintaining an adequate glycogen supply in both the muscles and the liver is imperative for sustained energy. For that reason, dates are best consumed shortly before, during or immediately following exercise. Other foods such as chlorophyll rich ones convert to glycogen as well but not as quickly as glucose, therefore making the easily-digestible, alkaline-forming date the ideal snack to fuel activity.

# Sample meal plan and recipes:

## BREAKFAST:

Toasted cereal with nut milk, fruit and yerba maté tea.

*To make nut milk:*
- *grind ¹/₂ cup of soaked nuts, seeds or both in blender (almonds, cashews, and hemp seeds work great; be creative)*
- *add ¹/₂ cup water; blend until smooth*
- *add ¹/₂ cup apple juice; liquefy*
- *add more water if desired*
- *Filter through a strainer if desired. (Personally, I like the unstrained texture.) Save the puree to spread on toast, add to soups, or whatever else you can think to do with it.*
- *for chocolate milk, mix in roasted carob powder*

## POST-WORKOUT SNACK:

Recovery pudding.

## SNACK:

Nutrient-rich shake.

## LUNCH:

Salad with lightly stir-fried extra-firm tofu. Yerba maté dressing and apple slices with hemp or almond butter.

**SNACK:**
Rejuvenator brownie (or nutrient-rich shake).

**DINNER:**
Raw soup.

As a general rule, most of the day's carbohydrates are consumed in the morning with modest amounts of protein. As the day progresses, that ratio shifts to consist primarily of protein, with a reduction in carbohydrates.

# Recipes:

The following are some examples of what you'll find in my full-length cookbook, to be completed in 2006.

### CHOCOLATE RECOVERY PUDDING

This pudding is easily digestible. It's the ideal 4:1 (carbohydrate to protein) ratio for optimized recovery.

| | |
|---|---|
| • *1/4 pound medium-firm tofu* | *- protein, calcium* |
| • *1 banana* | *- electrolytes* |
| • *1/2 pear* | *- natural sugar, fibre* |
| • *1/2 tbsp hemp oil* | *- EFAs* |
| • *1/2 tbsp cocoa powder* | *- natural flavour* |
| • *sprinkle sea salt* | *- sodium (lost in sweat)* |

Blend all ingredients together until reaching a consistent texture. Eat within 45 minutes after completing a workout.

## TOASTED APPLE CINNAMON CEREAL

This is an excellent, nutritionally balanced cereal. Unlike traditional cereals, this one has lots of fibre, complete protein, essential fatty acids and calcium.

| | |
|---|---|
| • 1 cup oats (uncooked) | - low glycemic carbohydrate |
| • 1/2 cup hemp protein powder | - protein, EFAs, vitamin E |
| • 1/2 cup flax seeds, ground | - omega 3, fibre, protein |
| • 1/2 cup sunflower seeds | - EFAs, alkalizing protein |
| • 1/2 cup un-hulled sesame seeds | - calcium, protein |
| • 1/2 cup almonds, diced | - EFAs, alkalizing protein |
| • 1/2 apple, diced | - pectin |
| • 1/4 cup hemp oil | - EFAs |
| • 1/4 cup molasses | - iron |
| • 2 tbsp apple juice | |
| • 1 1/2 tsp cinnamon | |
| • 1/4 tsp nutmeg | |
| • 1/4 tsp whole stevia leaf, dried and ground | - blood sugar regulator |
| • 1/4 tsp sea salt | - sodium |

Preheat oven to 250F. Mix all dry ingredients together. Blend liquid ingredients until reaching a consistent texture. Combine liquid and dry. Mix well. Spread on bake tray. Bake for 1 hour. Let cool; break up.

You'll notice that this cereal is toasted at a lower temperature than traditional granola. The reason for this is to preserve the essential fatty acids. Heating foods with essential fatty acids above 350F is not recommended, since the heat can convert EFAs to trans fats.

Keep refrigerated to greatly extend freshness.

*Fact: Un-hulled sesame seeds have a significantly better nutritional profile than their hulled counterparts. For example, they contain 700 percent more calcium.*

## Toasted ginger pear cereal

A blend of several high-quality protein sources, this cereal ensures all the amino acids are met in substantial amounts. With almond milk, this cereal is a complete meal. Each moderate-size serving contains about as much protein as three eggs.

| | |
|---|---|
| • 1 $^1$/$_2$ cups buckwheat | - low glycemic carbohydrate |
| • 1 cup green lentils, soaked | - protein |
| • 3/$_4$ cup pumpkin seeds | - iron, zinc |
| • $^1$/$_2$ cup hemp protein powder | - protein, EFAs, vitamin E |
| • $^1$/$_2$ cup ground flax seeds | - omega 3, fibre, protein |
| • $^1$/$_2$ cup un-hulled sesame seeds | - calcium, protein |
| • 1 tbsp ginger root, fresh | - natural anti-inflammatory, digestive aid |
| • 1 tsp cinnamon | |
| • $^1$/$_4$ hemp oil | - EFAs |
| • $^1$/$_4$ cup molasses | - iron |
| • 1 pear, medium | - natural sugar, fibre |
| • sprinkle sea salt | - sodium |
| • $^1$/$_2$ tsp stevia, dried whole leaf | - blood sugar regulator, sweetener |

Pre-heat oven to 250F. Blend hemp oil, molasses, half of the pear and finely chopped ginger together until smooth. I use a hand blender. Dice other half of the pear into small cubes. Mix all dry ingredients and diced pear together. Add all liquid ingredients and mix well. Spread evenly over two bake trays, about 1 cm thick. Bake for 1 hour to 1 $^1$/$_4$ hours, depending on preferred crispness. Let cool. Break into desired size pieces.

### Variations
Molasses can be substituted with either pure maple or rice syrup.

*Tip: Soak lentils overnight instead of cooking them before using in this recipe. They'll retain nutrients and digest more easily.*

## REJUVENATOR BROWNIES

A tasty nutrient-rich snack, these brownies are gluten free, alkaline and a good substitute for conventional brownies.

| | |
|---|---|
| • *1 cup brown rice flour* | *- alkalizing, gluten free* |
| • *$1/2$ cup water* | |
| • *$2/3$ cup roasted carob powder* | |
| • *$1/2$ cup pineapple pieces (cut to desired size)* | *- digestive aid* |
| • *$1/2$ cup ground flax* | *- omega 3, fibre, protein* |
| • *$1/2$ cup un-hulled sesame seeds, ground* | *- calcium, protein* |
| • *$1/2$ cup coconut milk* | *- selenium (antioxidant)* |
| • *$1/2$ cup chopped raw almonds* | *- EFAs, alkaline protein* |
| • *$1/2$ cup unsweetened pineapple sauce* | *- digestive aid* |
| *(blend pineapple pieces in processor)* | |
| • *$1/2$ cup shredded coconut* | *- selenium (antioxidant)* |
| • *$1/4$ cup raw cane sugar* | |
| • *1 tbsp baking powder* | |
| • *$1/2$ tsp sea salt* | *- sodium* |

For additional adrenal support and energy through nourishment, add 7.5 grams (about 1 tbsp) of maca along with an additional 2 tsp of water.

Preheat oven to 300F. Lightly oil bake pan. In a food processor, process $1/2$ cup pineapple pieces until it's consistent texture. Add the water and coconut milk and process until smooth. In a bowl, mix dry ingredients together, making sure no lumps remain. Combine wet and dry ingredients, mix well and pour into lightly greased bake pan. You will notice that the mixture is not as moist as traditional mixtures; this is because it will be baked at a lower temperature to preserve the EFAs. Bake for 1 hour, or until brownies start to pull away from the pan.

Keep refrigerated to greatly extend freshness.

## RAW SOUP

An excellent summer soup, packed with naturally occurring electrolytes and enzymes, 4,000 mg of omega 3 (same as $1/2$ lb of wild coho salmon) 13.5 mg of iron (same as 4 lb of beef), 85 mg of vitamin C (same as one orange), 325 mg of calcium (same as 1 $1/2$ cups of milk), 14 g of fibre (same as $1/2$ cup of bran cereal), and 28 g of raw, alkaline protein.

- *3 cups of water*
- *2 cups tightly packed spinach* — *iron, chlorophyll*
- *$1/2$ cup fresh parsley* — *digestive aid, iron, vitamin C*
- *$1/2$ avocado* — *vitamin K, EFAs*
- *2 tbsp hemp protein powder* — *complete, alkalizing protein*
- *2 tbsp pumpkin seeds, soaked* — *iron, zinc, enzymes*
- *1 tbsp hemp oil* — *EFAs*
- *$1/2$ tbsp ginger root, fresh* — *natural anti-inflammatory, digestive aid*
- *$1/4$ tsp whole stevia leaf powder* — *blood sugar regulator, sweetener*
- *1 tsp lemon juice* — *lowers glycemic index*
- *1 tsp (2.5 g) chlorella powder* — *vitamin B12, chlorophyll, nucleic acids*

Blend together (I use a hand blender).

*Fact: Vitamin C helps aid the absorption of iron. Consuming foods with high vitamin C content along with iron-rich ones will improve the body's ability to fabricate red blood cells. An adequate supply of red blood cells is imperative for the peak performance since they deliver oxygen to working muscles.*

*Fact: Ginger contains a high amount of a compound called zingibain, one of the most active constituents in enzymes. Zingibain is particularly valuable for the improved digestion of protein.*

## SESAME MISO SOUP

This alkalizing, calcium-and trace-mineral-rich soup provides natural-source electrolytes to help restore balance after exercise.

- 2 cups water
- 1/2 cup firm tofu — protein
- 2 tbsp un-hulled sesame seeds, ground — calcium, protein
- 1 tbsp miso paste (soy or rice) — vitamin K
- 1 tbsp tamari
- a few strips of dulse — electrolytes
- a medium scallion — vitamin K

Finely dice tofu and chop scallion. Heat water and mix with rest of ingredients.

### Variations
For a more intense flavour, lightly stir-fry the tofu and scallion in sesame seed oil, then add the tamari. Black sesame seeds are also a nice variation from the standard. Include 1 tbsp of hemp protein for added nutrition.

## PAPAYA GINGER SALAD DRESSING

An enzyme-packed, blood-boosting salad dressing.

- 1/2 cup papaya — vitamin A and C, digestive aid
- 1/4 cup hemp oil — EFAs
- 2 tbsp apple cider vinegar — detoxifier
- 1 tbsp lemon juice — lowers glycemic index, creates alkalinity
- 1 tbsp pumpkin seeds, soaked — iron, zinc
- 1 tsp ginger root, fresh — natural anti inflammatory, digestive aid
- sprinkle sea salt — sodium

Finley chop ginger and pumpkin seeds. Blend all ingredients. Flavour will be more 'even' if it's left to infuse overnight.

## Tofu lime curry

Protein rich and alkalizing, this electrolyte packed main course is filling yet easily digested. Also, with the addition of natural anti-inflammatory ingredients, soft tissue repair is enhanced.

- *1 cup extra firm tofu* — *protein, calcium*
- *1 cup coconut milk* — *electrolytes*
- *$1/_2$ large red onion* — *fibre*
- *$1 1/_2$ cups cauliflower* — *fibre*
- *1 cup broccoli flowers* — *vitamin A and C*
- *1 cup spinach* — *iron, chlorophyll*
- *1 tbsp ginger root, fresh* — *natural anti-inflammatory, digestive aid*
- *3 cloves garlic* — *blood thinner*
- *1 tbsp lime juice* — *lowers glycemic index, creates alkalinity*
- *$1/_2$ tsp curry* — *improves circulation*
- *$1/_2$ tsp turmeric* — *natural anti-inflammatory*
- *$1/_4$ chili pepper, finely sliced (or $1/_2$ tsp chilies dried)*
- *$1/_4$ tsp cumin* — *natural anti-inflammatory*
- *$1/_2$ cup fresh cilantro* — *digestive aid, iron, vitamin C*

Chop up vegetables. Cut onion lengthwise into slender strips. Spinach should be torn into bite size pieces. Put aside. Grate or finely chop the ginger and garlic. Heat pan to medium - high. Cut tofu into cubes. Stir-fry tofu with 1 tbsp of coconut oil or coconut butter (sesame seed oil will also work). Once nicely browned, add 1 tbsp soy sauce, stir-fry until it's all absorbed. Add the ginger and garlic. Turn heat down to low - medium. Add vegetables, curry, turmeric, chilies, cumin, and coconut milk. Put on lid. Let steam for 5 minutes. Add lime juice and cilantro.

Best served with sprouted quinoa or buckwheat. Traditional brown rice also works nicely.

*Fact: Coconut milk is the result of blending coconut meat with coconut water. During World War II, when IV solutions were out of supply, coconut water was substituted because of its high electrolyte content.*

## NUTRIENT-RICH SHAKE

Before I formulated Vega I made this shake daily. As you can see, it contains many of my favourite ingredients.

| | |
|---|---|
| • *3 cups water (or 2 cups water and 1 1/2 cups ice)* | |
| • *1 banana* | *- electrolytes* |
| • *1/2 cup blueberries* | *- antioxidants* |
| • *1/2 pear* | *- natural sugar, fibre* |
| • *1 tbsp hemp oil* | *- EAFs* |
| • *1 tbsp ground flax seeds* | *- omega 3, fibre* |
| • *2 tbsp hemp protein* | *- complete protein* |
| • *1 tsp (2.5 grams) maca, powdered form* | *- sterols, alkaloids glucosinolates* |
| • *1 tsp (2.5 grams) chlorella, powdered form* | *- vitamin B12, chlorophyll, nucleic acids* |
| • *250 mg dairy-free probiotics* | *- good bacteria* |

Blend together. For variety, add either a tablespoon of raw pumpkin or sunflower seeds. Raw carob powder is also a good addition. To complement the amino acid profile, add a tablespoon of pea or rice protein concentrate.

## YERBA MATÉ SALAD DRESSING

| | |
|---|---|
| • *2/3 cup balsamic vinegar* | *- detoxifier* |
| • *1/2 cup hemp oil* | *- EAFs* |
| • *1/3 cup water* | |
| • *2 tbsp yerba maté (dry)* | *- vitamins, minerals, enzymes* |
| • *1 clove garlic* | *- anti-bacterial, blood thinner* |
| • *1 tsp dried basil* | |
| • *1 tsp dried cilantro* | |
| • *1/2 tsp dried thyme* | |

Finely chop or grate garlic. Shake all ingredients together in a bottle. Let sit overnight to allow flavours to infuse and nutrients in yerba maté to be extracted.

## Vega sport drink

A synergistic blend of high-quality fuel, I designed this drink to be used during activity. The banana and dates supply the high-quality carbohydrate and Vega provides the staying power. Yerba maté further alkalizes and increases the amount of antioxidants and trace minerals. Dulse supplies the electrolytes.

- 3 cups water (to increase electrolyte content, substitute half for young coconut water)
- $1/2$ serving natural or chocolate Vega
- $1/4$ cup dates, fresh or soaked (about two large dates)
- $1/2$ banana
- 1 tsp yerba maté (grind to a fine powder using a coffee grinder)
- $1/4$ cup fresh mint leaves
- 1 tsp dulse flakes

Blend together. Makes two servings (375 ml each).

### Nutritional value per serving:
| | |
|---|---|
| Carbohydrate: | 29 g |
| Protein: | 8 g |
| Fat: | 5 g |

*Fact: Water from a young coconut is the original sport drink. Still commonly used in South America by athletes to replenish electrolytes, coconut water helps prolong hydration better than plain water.*

*Tip: For sustained energy and a reduction in recovery time, start sipping this drink about 90 minutes into a workout.*

## VEGA ENERGY PUDDING

A nutritionally balanced blend of easily digestible high-nutrient foods, Vega energy pudding is the ideal pre-exercise snack.

- *2 bananas*
- *1 cup blueberries*
- *1 serving (68 g) chocolate Vega*
- *$1/2$ cup almonds, soaked*
- *2 tsp ground yerba maté (grind to a fine powder using a coffee grinder)*
- *1 tsp lemon juice*
- *$1/4$ tsp sea salt*

Process everything in a food processor.

Makes two servings.

**Nutritional value per serving:**

| | |
|---|---|
| Carbohydrate: | 55 g |
| Protein: | 22 g |
| Fat: | 18 g |

Refrigerate unused portion.

**Fact:** *Citrus fruit such as lemons are an anomaly since they are acidic yet have an alkalizing effect on the body.*

**Tip:** *for lasting energy and elevated performance, try consuming this snack about 2 hours before your next workout. Also useful as whole food mid-afternoon snack, Vega energy pudding will provide a nutrient-packed boost.*

## VEGA STAMINA CEREAL

On mornings with time to spare I'll slice up a variety of fruit and combine it with soaked nuts, seeds and Vega. I'll pour a slightly watered down 1/2 serving of either chocolate or natural Vega on top. You can get creative with the combinations. I've listed the ingredients I use most often. Try combining whichever are appealing to you.

- *shredded coconut*
- *almonds, soaked*
- *sunflower seeds, soaked*
- *hemp seeds*
- *flax seeds, ground*
- *buckwheat*
- *sesame seeds*
- *raw or roasted carob powder*

- *banana*
- *papaya*
- *pineapple*
- *pear*
- *apple*
- *mango*
- *blueberries*
- *grated ginger*

Stir it all together in a bowl.

Eat like cereal.

*Fact: Papaya and pineapple contain digestive aids. Papain is found in papaya and bromelain in pineapple.*

*Fact: Soaking the nuts and seeds overnight will improve their nutritional value.*

*Tip: Try Vega on whole grain cereals for a complete breakfast or long-lasting snack.*

## VEGA ENERGY BARS

These bars are the healthiest and among the easiest and least time consuming to prepare. No cooking required. Only a food processor is needed.

| Berry Vega cranberry bars | Chocolate Vega blueberry bars |
| --- | --- |
| • 1 cup dates, fresh or soaked | • 1 cup dates, fresh or soaked |
| • 1 serving (65 g) berry Vega | • 1 serving (68 g) chocolate Vega |
| • 1/4 cup cranberries | • 1/4 cup blueberries |
| • 1/4 cup walnuts | • 1/4 cup walnuts |
| • 1/4 cup un-hulled sesame seeds | • 1/4 cup un-hulled sesame seeds |
| • 1/4 cup almonds | • 1/4 cup almonds |
| • 1/2 tsp lemon zest | • 1 tsp lemon juice |
| | • 1 tsp lemon zest |

Process all ingredients in a food processor until desired texture is reached. Remove mixture from processor and put on a clean surface.

Add to mixture:
- 1/2 - 1 cup oats (use buckwheat to make gluten free)
- 1/2 cup frozen cranberries or blueberries

Knead mixture to work in oats and berries. Form into a brick. Slice into desired bar size pieces. As the bars dry they become easier to handle.

Makes 12 x 50 g bars.

**Nutritional value per bar:**

| | |
| --- | --- |
| Protein: | 5 g |
| Fat: | 5 g |
| Carbohydrate: | 18 g |

*Tip: I suggest making a big batch at one time. I individually wrap each bar and store them in the freezer for when I'm on my way out. These bars will not freeze solid, resulting in the perfect bar for winter sports.*

# Strategies for success summarized

As you have learned, whole-food, plant-based nutrition can greatly alleviate a large portion of total stress. Stress is a word frequently used yet often not understood in its full capacity. As a result, I believe many symptoms stemming from stress get attention while the cause remains overlooked. Broken down into categories, stress is better understood. As with many problems, once understood, steps can then be taken to eliminate the source, thereby preventing its return.

*Following is a summary of principles that I have found most helpful:*

## DIETARY

- Make nutrient rich whole foods the cornerstone of the diet.
- Consume enough nutrients to support your activity level and the biological regeneration of your cells for a reduction of biological age.
- Meet nutritional needs by consuming nutrient dense whole foods as opposed to supplementing with tablets.
- Avoid denatured foods.
- Gain energy through nourishment, not stimulation.
- Increase energy by conserving it on digestion and assimilation, eat efficient foods.
- Reduce dependency on sugary, starchy foods – recalibrate.
- Reduce stress by meeting nutritional needs, not exceeding them.
- Eat a daily dose of chlorophyll rich foods.

- Hydrate adequately throughout the day
- Avoid roast nuts and seeds, choose raw, or better yet, sprouted
- Consume an easily digestible nutrient-rich shake daily to give the digestive system a break; further reducing overall stress.

## BEHAVIOURAL

- During the day, natural light is important.
- Don't take on more than you can handle. Be realistic.
- Know that to address a weakness is a strength.
- If you can't change it, don't try.
- Engage in production stress whenever desired.
- Better-quality sleep promotes the building of a healthier, stronger body.
- For optimum health, exercise the right amount for you.
- A happier person is a healthier person. Allow flexibility in your program.
- Treat your body well. Your cognitive ability will also benefit.
- If your body has symptoms, there's a cause, so find it.
- At the end of the day, darkness will aid recovery and improve sleep quality.

# The story behind Vega

I first experimented with a vegan diet in 1990. At the age of 15, not knowing the intricacies of what I was getting into, mistakes were made. Initially, I can attribute my interest in existing exclusively on plant-based foods to my self-conjured belief that it might improve athletic performance. I was wrong, at first.

In the beginning, I feasted on refined, denatured carbohydrates and manufactured fats to fulfil my seemingly insatiable appetite. Eating from the first onset of light until dark, I was having difficulty maintaining nourishment despite the fact that my stomach was full. Having trouble mustering energy to get through the day, my cognitive ability also became compromised.

An unmistakable decline in athletic performance caught the eye of my high school track coach. In addition, my teachers were less than enthused by the lethargy and impaired concentration that I began to exhibit. I needed encouragement, and I got it. Encouraged by many to start 'eating normally,' it was not the kind of advice I was looking for.

As a persistent 15-year-old, resistance to my plan seemed to lend it a certain allure. 'It can't be done' is what I was being told. 'You have to choose: do you want to be an athlete or a vegan?' This seemed to be popular opinion. In retrospect, I realize that lack of encouragement was exactly what I needed to fuel my curiosity. Could it be done? I decided to see if I could make it work.

I began to investigate. Medical journals, applied dietary studies and health and nutrition publications were my sources of choice. Initially there were not any studies to be found that supported exclusive plant-based nutrition for the athlete. However, there was also very little to discourage it! Fuelled by the lack of discouragement, I remained optimistic. That said, I realized that I'd have to be my own test subject and carefully track my findings – first hand research at its best.

Upon additional investigation, I learned that several nutrients of great importance, and commonly lacking for vegans, were deficient in my diet. This was a good start and just what I wanted to hear. I now had a reason for my malaise; the hardest part was behind me. I had identified the deficiencies: Complete protein, iron, omega-3 fatty acids, calcium and vitamin B12 were all lacking in my diet.

As a means to fulfilling my dietary shortcomings, I began making a blender drink with several of my newfound favourite foods. It was easy to do and it worked very well for me. Over time, the constant hunger, fatigue and poor recovery rate all dissipated. I was more than satisfied with what I had achieved. Now performing at a higher level, I felt as though my persistence and hard work had paid off. Several years passed and as they did my satisfaction turned into complacency. I was still performing well, but always believed that further gains could be made.

My interest in further improving athletic performance through diet was rekindled when I heard an ad on the radio for maca. "Maca has an amazing attribute—it can help reduce cortisol levels caused by stress," the announcer went on to say more but that's all I needed to investigate further since adrenal fatigue was a constant concern for me during periods of heavy training.

I researched maca thoroughly and found it was for real; certainly not a 'magic pill' or a cure for all problems, but a nutrient-dense whole food with a 'modern world' application. It helped to know native Peruvians had been taking maca for centuries for greater energy, strength and stamina and to this day it's still their #1 health food. I began adding the suggested daily teaspoon to my growing blender drink.

As a firm believer in the value of replenishment as apposed to stimulation for energy production, I knew that maca was the type of addition I had been looking for. Acknowledging the value of a balanced endocrine system from previous research, I knew that if I were able to rejuvenate my hormonal system, my energy levels would also improve. Extremely pleased with my discovery of maca, I wondered if there were other whole foods that could further improve health. The answer was yes.

My next great superfood addition was chlorella, a microscopic green algae from Japan. I was interested in it from the onset as a natural alternative to vitamin B12, but I found that it offered so much more. Its rich stores of protein, highly alkaline nature and unparalleled chlorophyll content made it my favourite green food. Furthermore, its unique Chlorella Growth Factor (CGF) offered amazing benefits in the area of cellular regeneration. Interesting to note, Japan, whose citizens have the longest life expectancy are also the greatest consumers of chlorella.

I began adding a teaspoon of chlorella to my ever-evolving daily blender drink. Not only did chlorella look good on paper, it actually delivered. Very pleased with the results, I could now eliminate the few remaining vitamin and mineral tablets that I had been taking. Vitamin B12 and calcium were the last to go at the hands of chlorella.

I am happy to report that by this time several studies and clinical trials had been conducted on plant-based nutrition. Many highly respected medical doctors, nutritionists, and dietary researchers were now encouraging the substitution of many plant-based products for animal ones.

## VEGA WAS BORN

Impressed with both the MacaSure brand of maca and ChlorEssence brand of chlorella that I had been using, I approached Sequel Naturals, the manufacturer, and met with the owner, Charles Chang. Starting from the beginning, I told Charles my story. I proposed the idea of combining my blender drink formula with MacaSure and ChlorEssence in a commercial version that anyone could take.

Since my blender drink formula had proven itself on a daily basis over the last eight years, it was clear that it was effective. Providing all the nutrition that a professional Ironman triathlete needed while maintaining a vegan diet spoke for itself. Charles liked the fact that I not only was able to 'exist' on a vegan diet, but actually thrive on one. Charles pondered the implications, "if this formula can fulfill the nutritional needs of a professional vegan athlete who doesn't take supplements and is pushing his body to the limit each day, imagine what could it do for the average person!"

Appreciating the obvious value, Charles was excited about the possibilities. Also a bit tentative because nothing like this had been replicated before, Charles wondered if it was possible. A great concept on paper, but could it be done? Charles and I committed ourselves to the necessary research and development. Over the course of about a year and a half, we answered all the questions earlier posed to us – by us.

Charles gave me complete control of the formulation process. 'I'm giving you a blank slate, go to it without compromise' he said. Exactly the words I wanted to hear. We spared no expense and Vega was made with the goal of replicating my proven blender drink as closely as possible. And thus, Vega was born.

*Of course the gains that many others and I have experienced with Vega could be replicated with sensible eating. The trouble is that sometimes it's not always convenient. Shortly before the launch of Vega, my blender drink had evolved to contain a synergistic blend of hemp protein, flax seeds, pea protein, rice protein, maca, chlorella, enzymes, pre and probiotics, as well as berries for antioxidants. When traveling or training long hours, making my blender drink had become tedious. Since the creation of Vega however getting top-rate nutrition has been greatly simplified.*

The launch of Vega was rewarding. Knowing it will help thousands of people achieve a better quality of life through improved health is tremendously satisfying.

## WHY VEGA WORKS

### *Healthy, convenient food for everyone and anyone*

The reason for my rapid fitness gains were due to the fact that I was simply recovering at a faster rate than previously. As a result I was able to train again sooner and harder, inevitably leading to a greater level of fitness in a shorter amount of time. Making the connection, it became apparent that expedited recovery was a result of nothing more than the removal of stress from my body. I saw the wide-spread implication. Having learned first hand that the body's response to stress is the same regardless of its source, I knew that Vega could help people curtail it and reap the benefits.

One of the most promising aspects of the formula was its potential to benefit a wide variety of people. Experienced first hand, stress rises when life gets busy. Yet the busier a person becomes the less time remains to prepare healthy food, most usually leading to the creation of a vicious circle. Sometimes referred to as the 'high achiever's paradox', this situation can lead to premature burnout. When good nutrition is most critical is the very time when it's usually gone without. Being too busy to prepare wholesome food, coupled with the integration of denatured convenience food options is a recipe for elevated stress.

Vega can help busy people reduce nutritional stress through providing nutrient-rich whole foods in a convenient and enjoyable form.

## ADDITIONAL ENERGY THROUGH CONSERVATION, NOT CONSUMPTION

Reducing the amount of energy expended on digestion, assimilation, and absorption allows for a greater net gain than traditional foods can offer. Since Vega contains natural digestive enzymes, is alkaline forming and is in liquid form, energy is conserved in its utilization. As you read earlier, conservation is another way to obtain more energy. Efficiency in spending becomes the determining factor as to how much energy we have. By consuming Vega, a large part of the initial energy boost noticed can be attributed to conservation not consumption, and of course not to stimulation.

## IMPROVED PERFORMANCE THROUGH REJUVENATION, NOT STIMULATION

The second way in which Vega provides more energy is by nourishing the adrenal glands and the endocrine system as a whole. By requiring fewer resources to utilize its nutrients, Vega allows the body to spend its energy elsewhere. As a result the body can now put more of its resources into improving immune system function, recovering from exercise and coping with stress.

By spending energy on stress tolerance, cortisol levels become reduced. Once cortisol levels decline, the body is better able to maintain lean muscle and shed fat. In addition, the ability to fall asleep and quickly slip into the deep regenerative phase known as Delta is only possible when cortisol levels are low. Once the body is able to spend a greater amount of time in the Delta phase of sleep, effectively improving sleep efficiency, waking up will be easier.

Feeling rested and restored will be the result and, as such the desire to stimulate by consuming sugary, starchy and caffeine-containing foods will be reduced. As this process transpires, it will set off a complementary circle—a positive chain of events. Some describe the effect this way: 'When I sleep I'm more asleep, consequently when I'm awake I'm more awake.' The line between being asleep and being awake becomes more starkly defined, certainly a deviation from our current cultural norm.

Now that the desire to 'borrow' energy from sugar, starch and caffeine has begun to dissipate, sleep will continue to improve since the cortisol raising attributes of sugar, starch and caffeine will have been further reduced.

## FIVE SYNERGISTIC SOURCES OF PROTEIN

By synergistically combining five protein sources, I found that my ability to recover improved dramatically. Improved recovery is, of course, an indication that stress has been relived from the body. Amino acid levels vary in all protein sources. By synergistically selecting complementary sources and amounts, we can achieve what is referred to as a 'flat line profile.' An indicator that all amino acids are being met in substantial quantities, the 'flat line profile' of properly combined amino acids is indicative of a broadspectrum source of protein.

Found predominantly in hemp, edestin is an easily digestible form of protein. Beneficial for the structural integrity of our cell's DNA, edestin more closely resembles human protein than any other in the plant kingdom.

The branch chain amino acids leucine, isoleucine and valine are prevalent in hemp protein. Essential for the repair and building of lean muscle tissue these branch chain amino acids are also an integral part of maintaining a healthy metabolic rate.

Hemp protein by itself is complete, but there is still room for improvement. Relatively low in the essential amino acid tryptophan, hemp protein is nicely complemented by the addition of rice protein. Naturally prominent in rice protein, tryptophan helps the body fabricate serotonin. With more readily available serotonin in the system, mood will be elevated, resulting in fewer sugar and starch cravings.

Relatively hard to find in the plant kingdom, the amino acid lysine is exceptionally high in yellow pea protein. An essential amino acid, lysine is a critical factor in the production of enzymes, antibodies and hormones. The body's ability to maintain correct nitrogen balance and absorb calcium is also reliant on the presence of lysine in the diet. During times of augmented stress, the maintenance of lean muscle tissue is assisted by the consumption of lysine rich foods.

Not only complete, this combination is complementary and synergistic, it is structured better than any single protein source can ever be. As a direct result from the 'flat line' amino acid profile, I noticed immediate gains in strength and lean muscle retention, even during times of elevated stress. The desire to consume more food dissipated as well, leaving me leaner.

## No common allergens

A standard practice in naturopathic medicine is to first eliminate all sources of common allergens from the diet. This is a logical way to determine if the patient has an allergy or sensitivity to commonly eaten foods that can produce a wide range of symptoms. Ranging from mild flu like symptoms, to headaches, difficulty sleeping, bloating and fatigue, food sensitivities are becoming increasingly common. Since foods such as wheat, dairy products, soy, corn, and gluten have become so common in our food chain, the body can develop an intolerance, which often results in the manifestation of symptoms.

In my opinion food allergies are not a major problem because they become evident immediately upon consumption. There's no mistaking it, the symptoms are instant. Stop consuming the problem-forming food and the problem is solved. Conversely, food sensitivities can be extremely difficult to ascertain, therefore they are more difficult to eliminate. The symptoms of a food sensitivity might not become evident for a few days or a week after consumption, making its exact origin difficult to trace.

For a few years in a row I had what I thought to be a bad case of hay fever each spring. A logical possibility since pollen counts increase that time of year therefore, I didn't think much of it. The following year, after learning more about food sensitivities, I tried eliminating all common allergens from my diet. As springtime arrived this time, surprise—no hay fever. Confirmed later, the congestion that I had previously exhibited was due to my sensitivity to corn, and not to rising pollen counts. Once spring arrived I began cycling more, therefore consumed a larger quantity of a so-called endurance enhancing sport drink. The first ingredient was maltodextrin, a cheap sugar derivative made from corn, and as I found out, the precipitator of my hay fever-like symptoms.

## ALKALINE FORMING

It amazes me how little attention the value of balanced pH has garnered from the mainstream medical world. In my opinion, positive acid/alkaline balance is one of the most important factors for improving athletic performance. By disregarding this factor, sport supplement manufactures have significantly reduced the effectiveness of their products.

After a hard training session the body will have increased its acidity due to lactic acid accumulation caused by muscle contractions. For recovery to be expedited, alkalizing foods, especially those rich in chlorophyll, need to be consumed soon after. Protein must also be consumed to help repair broken down muscle tissue. Many sport supplements touted as post-work-out recovery agents contain highly processed, manufactured proteins, usually in the form of denatured isolates, which are acid forming. If consumed soon after a workout they will certainly fulfil the body's need for protein, but completely neglect its requirement for pH balancing.

The paradox is this: most protein sources are highly acid forming, yet the majority of highly alkaline forming foods are low in protein. As I found, this can be overcome, if the protein sources are chosen carefully. Raw, unprocessed, natural, hemp protein powder, for example, contains about 50% protein, yet is considerably less acid forming than common soy or whey protein products. Hemp's higher pH level can be attributed in part to chlorophyll content, responsible for its green colour. Chlorella is another one, almost 70% protein and highly alkalizing. Whole micro-milled flax seeds, enzymes, stevia, probiotics, and the berry complex contained in Vega also help increase its alkalinity.

By consuming natural, non-denatured proteins after my training sessions I noticed a vast improvement in my ability to fight infection, proving my immune system's effectiveness had greatly improved. My body no longer created a safe haven for bacteria, viruses or disease. In addition, my protein requirements were being met so I was able to maintain and build lean muscle tissue and strength.

For more extensive information about Vega please contact the manufacturer Sequel Naturals directly at:

1-866-839-8863
www.myvega.com

# Afterword

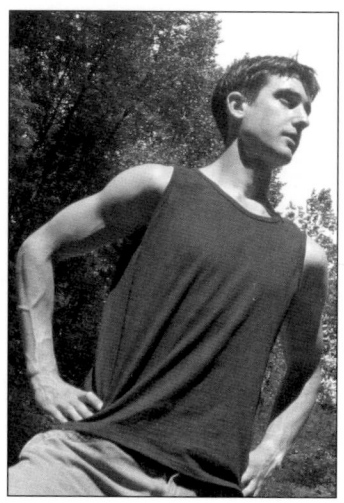

Throughout the last 14 years I have learned how to perform at a high level in one of the world's most demanding sports, while exclusively on a plant-based diet. I know that a strict vegan way of life is not for everyone but believe me, incorporating more plant-based foods into your current diet will make a substantial difference. Apply as few or as many of the principles outlined in this book as you are comfortable with, every bit counts.

Congratulations for taking the initiative to improve your health and performance through my nutritional stress reduction program. Obviously by reading this book you have made a decision to empower yourself with knowledge. Now, armed with knowledge, all that's left to do is apply it and reap the rewards.

Whatever you choose to do with your newly acquired vitality, I wish you all the best.

To your ambitions,

*Brendan*

Brendan Brazier

# Appendix

## VEGA / MACA / CHLORELLA

### Sequel Naturals

Makers of MacaSure brand premium quality gelatinized organic maca and ChlorEssence brand high growth factor chlorella, and of course Vega.

1-866-839-8863
info@sequelnaturals.com
www.sequelnaturals.com

## HEMP

### Living Harvest and Manitoba Harvest hemp foods

As you have read I'm a big proponent of hemp food for both human and environmental health. Both Living Harvest and Manitoba Harvest grow premium quality hemp, turning it into hemp food in the form of raw protein powder, seed, oil, and flour, all top quality. Never grown with herbicides or pesticides Living Harvest and Manitoba Harvest are both first-rate models of sustainable agriculture. Both of these companies use a milling process that preserves all the natural goodness of the plant, further increasing its food value.

Living Harvest:
1-888-690-3958
info@livingharvest.com
www.livingharvest.com

Manitoba Harvest:
1-800-665-4367
info@manitobaharvest.com
www.manitobaharvest.com

## WHOLE GRAIN CEREAL / FLAX

### Nature's Path Foods

Nature's Path is the largest producer of 100% organic hot and cold cereals, manna bread and other top quality grain foods. Using only premium ingredients, never genetically modified, Nature's Path cereal has been a part of my high performance diet since the early 1990's. Nature's Path also has a line of organic whole flax seeds that I use in many of my recipes. As a pioneer in organic agriculture on a large scale, Nature's Path has encouraged many other manufactures to follow in its eco-friendly footsteps.

1-888-808-9505
consumer_services@naturespath.com
www.naturespath.com

## TOFU

### Sunrise Soya Foods

Makers of high quality tofu. Sunrise Soya Foods produces a line of tofu called Soyganic, made from 100% organic, non-genetically modified, Canadian grown soy beans.

1-800-661-2326
consumer-info@sunrise-soya.com
www.sunrise-soya.com

## YERBA MATÉ

### *Aviva Ltd.*

Rich in chlorophyll and antioxidants, Aviva yerba maté is a health-boosting plant, ideal for increasing sustainable energy and promoting recovery. Aiding digestion and carrying an alkaline balance, Aviva air-dried yerba maté is never roasted, preserving its full array of nutrients.

Since Aviva only uses wild harvest yerba maté you can be assured that it is grown with the jungle, not instead of the jungle, helping to preserve sustainable agriculture. Wild harvest yerba maté is grown under the tall jungle canopy, protecting the soft subtle leaves from the harsh South American sun, allowing them to remain edible. Edible leaves, another reason why I use Aviva yerba maté in several of my recipes.

1-877-255-1473
contact@yerba-mate.com
www.yerba-mate.com

## SEA VEGETABLES

### *Maine Coast Sea Vegetables*

Sustainabley harvested and certified organic, Maine Coast provides several varieties of premium quality raw sea vegetables.

207-565-2907
info@seaveg.com
www.seaveg.com

## Eco-friendly clothing and shoes

### *Of The Earth Clothing*

Makers of stylish environmentally friendly clothing. Of The Earth uses hemp, organic cotton, linen (from the flax plant), and soy fabrics to create premium quality clothing while practicing sustainable agriculture.

1-877-683-4367
retail@oftheearth.com
www.oftheearth.com

### *Hemptown Clothing Inc.*

Makers of environmental friendly hemp clothing.

1-866-436-7869
info@hemptown.com
www.hemptown.com

### *Shoes with Souls*

Stylish yet sustainable. Shoes with Souls makes a wide variety of eco-friendly, synthetic fabric shoes.

858-653-3741
info@shoeswithsouls.com
www.shoeswithsouls.com

# References

Adlercreutz, H. Western diet and Western diseases: some hormonal and biochemical mechanisms and associations. Scand J Clin Lab Invest 1990;201(suppl):3-23

Bravo, L. Polyphenol: Chemistry, dietary sources, metabolism, and nutritional significance. Nutr Rev 1998;56(II): 317-33.

Burke, E.R. Optimal Muscle Recovery, New York: Avery Publishing Group, 1999.

Cao, G., et al. Antioxidant capacity of tea and common vegetables. J Agric Food Chem 1996;4:34 26-31.

Cao, G., et al. Increases in Human plasma antioxidant capacity after consumption of controlled diets high in fruit and vegetables. Am J Clin Nutr 1998;68:1081-7.

Colgan, M. Optimum Sports Nutrition. New York: Advanced Research Press, 1993.

Colgan, M. Essential Fats. Vancouver: Apple Publications, 1998.

Colgan, M. The New Nutrition. Vancouver: Apple Publishing, 1996.

Colgan, M. Hormonal Health. Vancouver: Apple Publishing, 1995.

Colgan, M. Protein for Muscle and Strength, Vancouver: Apple Publications, 1998.

Conrad, C. Hemp for Health: The Medicinal and Nutritional uses of Cannabis Sativa. Inner Traditions Intl Ltd, 1997.

Cordain, L. The Paleo Diet: Lose Weight and Get Healthy by Eating the Food Your Were Designed to eat, Wiley 7 son, New York, 2001.

Coulstron, A.M. The role of Dietary fats in plant-based diets. Am J Nutr 1999;70(suppl):512S-5S.

Coyne, L.L. Fat Won't Make You Fat. Fish Creek Publishing, 1998

De Kloet, E.R. 'Corticosteroids, Stress, and Aging,' Annals of New York Academy of Sciences, 663 (1992), 358.

Erasmus, U. Fats and Oils. Vancouver: Alive Books, 1986

Fabris, N, et al, (eds). Physiopathological Processes of Aging, New York: Academy of Sciences, 1992

Ferrandiz, M.L., et al. Anti-inflammatory activity and inhibition of arachidonic acid metabolism by flavonoids. Agents Actions 1991;32:283-8.

Giese, AC. Living With Our Sun's Ultraviolet Rays. Plenum Pr. 1976

Graci, S. The Power of Super Foods: 30 Days that will Change Your Life, Toronto: Prentice Hall Canada, Inc, 1997.

Green, MB. Eating Oil: Energy Use in Food Production. Westview Press. 1978

Hall, JV. Valuing the health benefits of clean air. Science 1992;255:812-816.

Hart, A. Adrenaline and Stress / the Exciting New Breakthrough That Helps You Overcome Stress Damage. Word Publishing; Revised edition July 1995.

Hayflick, L. How and why we Age. New York: Ballantine, 1994.

Holick, M.F. Vitamin D: the underappreciated D-lightful hormone that is important for skeletal and cellular health. Curr Opin Endocrinal Diabetes 2002;9:87-98.

Howell E, Murray M. Enzyme Nutrition. Lotus Press. 1986.

Hunter, Beatrice T. The Natural Foods Primer. New York: Simon and Schuster, 1972

Joseph, J.A., et al. Oxidative stress production and vulnerability in aging: putative nutritional implications for intervention. Mech Ageing Dev 2000;31;116(2-3):141-53

Kikuzaki, H., Kawasaki, Y., and Nakatani, N. Structure of antioxidative compounds in ginger. ACS Sympisium series. 547:237-243. 1994.

King, B.J: Fat Wars Action Planner. Wiley & Sons, Canada, 2003.

King, B.J. and M.A. Schmidt. Bio-Age: Ten Steps to a Younger You, Macmillan Canada, 2001.

Kraemer, W.J. et al. 'Effects of Heavy-Resistance Training on Hormonal Response Patterns in Younger and Older Men,' J Appl Physiol, 1999, 87, no. 3: 982-92.

Krebs-Smith, S.M., et al. The effects of variety in food choices on dietary quality. J Am Diet Assoc 1987;87(7):896-903.
Kushi, M., and A. Kushi. Macrobiotic Diet. New York: Japan Publication, 1985

Kusnecov, A and B.S. Rabin. 'Stressor-Induced Alterations of Immune Function: Mechanisms and Issues,' International Archives of Allergy and Immunology 105 (1994), 108.

Ley, BM. Maca: Adaptogen and Hormonal Regulator, Detroit Lakes: BL Publications. 2003.

Ley, BM. Chlorella: The Ultimate Green Food, Detroit Lakes: BL Publications. 2003.

Lardinois, C.K. 'The Role of Omega-3 Fatty Acids on Insulin Secretion and Insulin Sensitivity,' Med Hypotheses, 1997, 24 (3): 243-8.

Leibowitz, S.,et al. 'Insulin Plays role in Controlling Fat Craving,' News from the Rockefeller University, New York, NY, 1995.

Levine, S. and H. Ursin, 'What is Stress?' in S. Levine and H. Ursin, eds., Psychobiology of Stress (New York: Academic Press), 17.

Loche, S. E. 'Stress, Adaptation, and Immunity: Studies in Humans,' General Hospital Psychiatry 4 (1982), 49-58.

Messina, M. Legumes and Soybeans: overview of their nutritional profiles and health effects. Am J Clin Nutr 1999;70(3suppl):439S-50S.

Nick, G.L. Detoxification properties of low-dose phytochemical complexes found within select vegetables. JANA 2002;5(4):34-44.

Nuernberger, P. Freedom from Stress. Honesdale, Pa.: Himalayan International Institute, 1981

Pert C, Molecules of Emotions: Why you Feel the Way you Feel. New York: Tochstone, 1999, 22-23.

Perricone, N. The Wrinkle Cure: Unlock the Power of Cosmeceuticals for Supple, Youthful Skin. Warner Books, 2001

Pieri C, et al. Melatonin as an effective antioxidant. Arch Gerontol Geriatr, 1995;20:159-165.

Prasad, C. 'Food, Mood and Health: A Neurobiologic Outlook,' Braz J Med Biol Res, Dec 1998, 31, no.12 :1517-27.

Quillin, P. Beating Cancer with Nutrition. Tulsa, OK: Nutrition Times Press, 1994.

Rankin, J.W. 'Role of Protein in Exercise,' Clin Sports Med, 18(3): 499-511, 1999.

Reiter, RJ. Oxygen radical detoxification processes during aging: the functional importance of melatonin. Aging Clin Exp Res, 1995;7:340-351.

Richardson JH, Palmenton T, Chenan H. The effect of calcium on muscle fatigue. J Sports Med 1980;20:149.

Robinson, R. The Hemp Manifesto: 101 ways that hemp can save our world. Inner Traditions Intl Ltd, 1997.

Schmidt, M.A. Smart Fats, Berkeley: North Atlantic Books, 1997.

Sears, B. The Anti-Aging Zone, New York, NY: HarperCollins, Inc., 1999.

Seeman, T.E. and B. S. McEwen, 'Impact of Social Environmental Characteristics on Neuroendocrine Regulation,' Psychosomatic Medicine 58 (September-October 1996), 462.

Simopoulos, A.P. Essential Fatty Acids in Health and Chronic Disease. Am J Clin Nutr 1990;70(suppl):560S-9S.

Somer, E. and N.L. Snyderman. Food and Mood: The complete guide to Eating Well and Feeling Your Best: Owl Books, 1999

Stanitski, C. Air pollution affects exercise performance. Clinics in Sports Medicine. 1986;4:725-726'

Stoll, A.L. The Omega 3 Connection. New York: Simon & Schuster, 2001.

Teitelbaum, J.E, et al. Nutritional impact of pre- and probiotics as protective gastrointestinal organisms. In: Annual Review of Nutrition, vol. 22, 2002. McCormick, D.B., Bier, D., Cousins, R.J., eds., Palo Alto, CA: Annual Reviews,107-38.

Vandler, AJ. Nutritional Stress and Toxic Chemicals. Ann Arbor: University Pres, 1981

Viru, A. Hormones in Muscular Activity. Boca Raton, Fl: CRC Press, 1985.

Wilson JL. Adrenal Fatigue: The 21st-Century Stress Syndrome. Smart Publications. 2002.

Wood R. The New Whole Foods Encyclopedia: A Comprehensive Resource for Healthy Eating. Penguin USA. July 1999.

Wright S. Essential fatty acids and the skin. Br J Derm 125:503-515, 1991.

Wurtman, J.J. and S.Suffers. 'The Serotonin Solution', Ballantine Books, 1997.

Van Cauter, E., and G Copinschi. 'Interrelationships Between Growth Hormone and Sleep.' Growth Hormone IGH Res Supplement. April 2000. B:S57-62.

Youdim, KA. Martin A, Joseph JA. 'Essential Fatty Acids and the brain: possible health implications'. Int J Dev Neurosci 18:383-99, 2000

Young. V.R., and P.L. Pellett. 'Plant Proteins in Relation to Human Protein and Amino Acid Nutrition.' American Journal of Clinical Nutrition 59 (1994): 1203-1212S.